THE POWER OF YOGA FOR MEN

A beginner's guide to building strength, mental clarity and emotional fitness

BLOOMSBURY SPORT
Bloomsbury Publishing Plc
50 Bedford Square, London, WC1B 3DP, UK
29 Earlsfort Terrace, Dublin 2, Ireland

First published in Great Britain 2022

A catalogue record for this book is available from the British Library
Library of Congress Cataloguing-in-Publication data has been applied for

ISBN: PB: 978-1-4729-8930-7; eBook: 978-1-4729-8929-1; ePdf: 978-1-4729-8928-4

2 4 6 8 10 9 7 5 3 1

Design by Lee-May Lim
Typeset in JohnstonITC by Lee-May Lim
Printed and bound in China by Toppan Leefung Printing

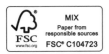

To find out more about our authors and books visit www.bloomsbury.com and sign up
for our newsletters.

THE POWER OF YOGA FOR MEN

A beginner's guide to building strength, mental clarity and emotional fitness

CALEB JUDE PACKHAM & JAROD CHAPMAN

BLOOMSBURY SPORT

LONDON • OXFORD • NEW YORK • NEW DELHI • SYDNEY

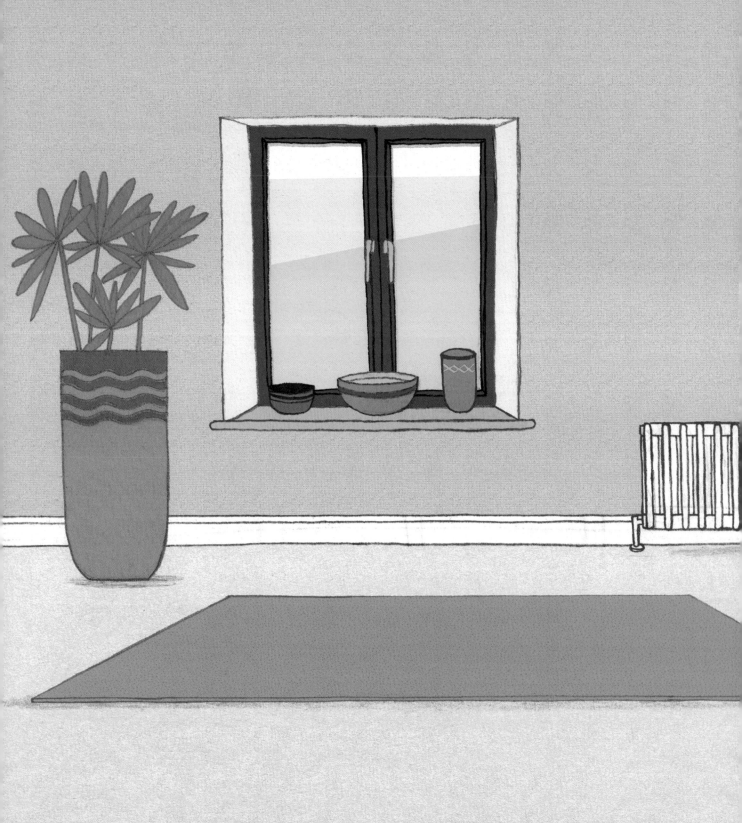

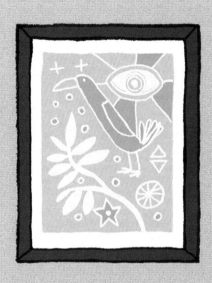

CONTENTS

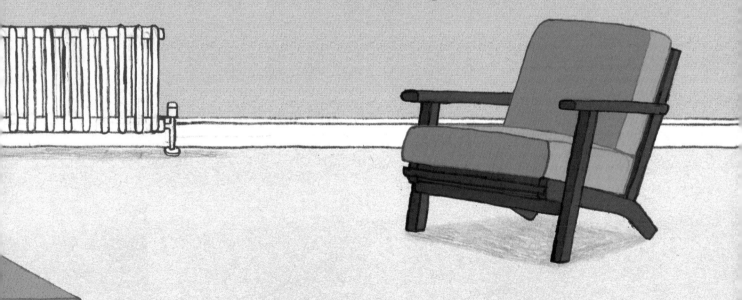

WELCOME TO THE MAT

If you've picked up this book, chances are you can't remember the last time (if ever) you did a yoga class or even thought about it. You can't touch your toes, or wrap your arms behind your back, nor can you meditate (nor have you tried) because both your mind and your diary are far too full for that.

Or maybe you're that guy who's done a yoga class or two, but you've been put off by your inflexibility. You feel uncoordinated and unbalanced, which makes you frustrated. You think; to heck with it, I'm gonna go play football and tear a hamstring instead.

But the thing is, there's a shift happening. And you know it. More and more men are stepping on to the yoga mat, accessing its power in body, mind and spirit. They're becoming stronger, more flexible, mentally clear and emotionally attuned.

So here you are. Willing to try something new. Ready to work on yourself. You might be feeling a little unsure, or maybe sceptical. And that's okay.

As the authors of this book, we welcome you to the mat. This is where your yoga journey begins. You're about to discover the incredible power of this ancient practice, its origins, and its applications for a man in today's world – and it won't be what you expect!

WHAT IS YOGA?

Yoga = union.

The word 'yoga' comes from the Sanskrit word 'yuj', which means to join together.

Yoga is the union of breath and body, mind and spirit.

It's an ancient practice with modern relevance; a fusion of East and West; a physical practice and an art form; a philosophy and a lifestyle.

Yoga teaches us that through breath, movement, sound and stillness we can quieten our mind and expand our awareness of ourselves and our surroundings.

On their own the yoga postures, or 'asanas', will improve physical strength, flexibility, balance and spinal health. Yet it's when we practise yoga regularly and with intention that we can truly cultivate the intelligence and intuition, sensitivity and wisdom that is so transformational.

Yoga is about getting to know yourself better. It can provide a much-needed source of calm during times of adversity and struggle. It can offer stillness and vitality, comfort and challenge. When one man works on himself it inspires another to do the same, rippling outwards, until the world is filled with pretty awesome men.

As you become more emotionally intelligent and responsive, your ability to nurture yourself and others will grow and develop. This makes life a whole lot more fulfilling, both on and off the mat.

If you're not convinced yet, that's okay. This isn't about brainwashing, but about practice. All we ask is that you try, often, and without cynicism, to unroll your mat and do some yoga. The rest will happen, breath by breath by breath.

BUSTING THE MYTHS

We know lots of men – even our friends! – who have misconceptions about yoga; who it's for and what it involves. We thought we'd set the record straight.

MYTH 1: YOGA IS JUST FOR WOMEN

This is one of the biggest myths a lot of guys have stuck in their heads. When in fact, throughout yoga's 5000-year history, it has been predominately men who have practised and passed on the lineage.

As yoga exploded across the West in the 1960s, it was women who embraced this movement, leaving us guys behind. Now it's our time to catch up!

MYTH 2: IT'S NOT A PROPER WORKOUT

If you think yoga is just stretching on a mat, think again. Yoga will test your strength, endurance and cardiovascular system with an intensity that's on a par with many a gym workout. Also, if you're a guy who has never done a proper workout in your life, yoga is a great place to start.

MYTH 3: YOU'RE NOT FLEXIBLE ENOUGH

Well, that's the reason to do yoga, not to avoid it.

MYTH 4: YOU CAN'T DO IT!

Maybe you're worried about embarrassing yourself in front of others. It's time to let that go. Yoga is not about judgement. No one cares if you can't wrap yourself up in Dragonfly Pose. With time and perseverance you will do it – or not – because at the end of the day it doesn't really matter, just as long as you're doing the practice.

MYTH 5: YOGA IS A RELIGION

While historically associated with Hinduism, Buddhism and Jainism, yoga is not a religion. You can belong to any faith, or not (yes, atheists, we're speaking to you) and still reap the benefits of devotion to your practice.

MYTH 6: YOU HAVE TO BE VEGAN TO DO YOGA

No, you don't. Although the yogic belief system certainly encourages a non-harming lifestyle, which includes not eating any animals, there are no hard and fast rules. You can eat what you like and still practise yoga.

MYTH 7: YOGA TAKES UP TOO MUCH TIME

One of the great things about yoga is that it takes up as much time as it takes up space. All you need is a yoga mat and the discipline to do it. And remember, 30 minutes of scrolling on social media could be 30 minutes on the mat. Now that's real connection.

MYTH 8: ALL YOGA IS THE SAME

Yogic practices have evolved over time, just as humans have. Today there's a myriad of different forms to explore. There's slow and meditative practices; dynamic, strong, physical practices; there's breath-work, chanting and free movement. Put it this way, you'll never get bored.

WHY YOU NEED THIS PRACTICE IN YOUR LIFE

YOGA HELPS TAME THE RESTLESS, ANXIOUS MIND

Anxiety is one of the biggest men's mental health issues today, and it's often suffered in silence. Sometimes people don't even realise they're experiencing it; it's become such a normal part of their everyday life. Guys, in particular, have been taught to be strong and stoic. But sometimes we are breaking on the inside. If this sounds like you, then taking up yoga will help. You're on the right path, we promise.

The power of yoga can be experienced immediately. As you move, as you breathe – as you figure out where to put your foot, your hand, your focus – yoga channels your mind away from anxious thoughts and into your body.

YOGA HELPS YOU KISS INSOMNIA GOODNIGHT

Insomnia literally does a man's head in (and often his partner's too). As anyone who has suffered it will know, it leaves you feeling moody, foggy-headed and ultimately exhausted.

If the underlying cause of your insomnia is burnout, stress or anxiety, then a regular yoga practice, including breath-work and meditation, will help you develop the ability to quieten the internal chatter of your mind and to relax your body too. These techniques, over time, will assist you into deep, restorative sleep.

YOGA HELPS YOU GET IT UP

One in five. That's the number of men who are known to suffer with Erectile Dysfunction. It's probably more, when you take into account the men who are suffering but don't admit it. The assumption is that this is a middle-aged man's issue. And that assumption is incorrect. In fact, guys in their 30s, even their 20s, can suffer from ED.

So how does yoga help? As with insomnia, a lot of ED causes are psychological, such as anxiety, stress and depression. Getting on the yoga mat every day can help pull you out of these negative thought patterns. And forget the Viagra – later on we'll show you some specific yoga techniques to increase blood flow to the penile arteries. The combination of a relaxed mind and healthy circulation restores sexual vitality and confidence.

YOGA HELPS YOU WALK THE BLACK DOG

Let's put paid to the commonplace notion that men don't suffer with mental health problems every bit as much as women do. Very sadly, and probably because we're slower to ask for help, we also make up three quarters of the suicidal deaths that take place every year.

Scientific studies have proven yoga to be a powerful treatment for depression as it literally gets you up and into your body, releasing feel-good chemicals and helping you to put a distance between the negative, self-defeating aspects of your mind and the rest of your being. The focused and controlled movements of the practice strengthen your mind–body connection, while the meditative element brings you into the present moment, which helps clear your mind.

YOGA HELPS YOU HEAL FROM BURNOUT

Work, family, responsibilities, commitments (and even more work) can slowly erode you to the edge of exhaustion. Sometimes you may not even realise you're burned out until the stress takes its toll physically, mentally and emotionally, leaving you feeling empty and depleted.

Taking time out for yoga helps relieve the impact of long-term exhaustion by reducing cortisol (a stress hormone), boosting immunity, increasing circulation and restoring energy. As yoga teaches you to slow down and live in the present moment, priorities fall into place and positivity is reignited.

YOGA HELPS BOOST CONFIDENCE

The need to fit in, and to measure up to certain supposedly masculine standards, often makes us guys feel insecure. As men, we're expected to be independent, powerful, the leader of the team. On top of that, we're apparently supposed to have big biceps, big pecs and washboard abs.

Yoga teaches authentic confidence that starts within and radiates out. It gives you strength and clarity of mind, which enables you to have a healthy sense of yourself. You don't get caught up with other people's negativity and you don't care about having big biceps because you're fit, supple and yoga strong.

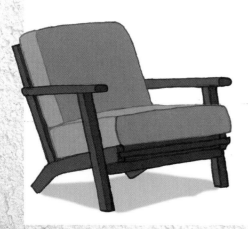

Rob's story

Rob joined the Royal Marines aged 16. Head shaved, boots on, he was surrounded by older men who showed him how to think, behave and endure. At first, it was exhilarating. Rob was filled up with military grit. The camaraderie, the sense of purpose.

There was never a dull moment. But also never a moment to breathe. During his time in active service, Rob lived in a persistent state of high alert, ever ready for battle or crisis. His training sessions were always gruelling, and not considered a success unless they left him beaten, on the floor, gasping for breath with muscles burning. Away from his family for nine months of every year, he learned to ignore his emotional needs and to switch off his body's pleas for calm and moderation. For years on end, Rob continued like this, able to withstand the most extreme physical and mental pressure without so much as a full exhale.

But even the most resilient, high-octane men can't keep going like this forever. Having been selected to be commander of a successful and significant operation, Rob was awarded the Distinguished Service Cross in 2015. It should have been a time of great pride and celebration, and yet, under the surface, he was struggling. When his marriage took a downturn and a subordinate took their own life, Rob's armour finally cracked. Even the man who had prided himself on his ability to endure (and endure and endure) had reached his limit. A warrior, yes, but also human.

Finally, after years of fighting (not just other people, but also himself), Rob did the one thing that he was trained never, ever to do. It was also the most courageous thing, under the circumstances, requiring humility, insight and trust. He visited the doctor and surrendered. Admitting that he could no longer function in the same way, and feeling exhausted beyond belief, Rob found himself unable to contain his tears. Next thing he knew, he was assigned to a recovery troop, a place where regular yoga was offered, and encouraged.

Curious, and with nothing much to lose, Rob hit the mat. He was surprised, almost immediately, by how challenging it was. He found it hard to be present, and his body was stiff in the extreme. Through regular practice, however, he felt his body soften and anxiety reduce. Slowly and safely, Rob began, through yoga, to release the physical and emotional trauma that had been holding him hostage.

Every day now, Rob practises yoga. This includes breathing exercises, asana practice and meditation. Inspired to teach the power of yoga to others, he recently became a fully certified yoga instructor, and spreads the message to other men. His story is one of true yogic transformation.

YOGA IS STRENGTH

You might already know that yoga strengthens the mind. So, let's talk about how it also strengthens your body.

The physical practice of yoga is a combination of holding static postures and performing dynamic movements connected to breath. This seamless transition from posture to posture, known as the 'vinyasa', requires you to support your body weight in relation to gravity as you move through your full range of motion.

Yoga is functional training. It strengthens and develops your body to healthily perform your daily activities, improving your balance, posture, muscular endurance and flexibility. The more you practise, the stronger you become in everything you do; walking, running, sitting, playing sport, etc.

Yoga not only strengthens your muscles and joints but also your energy systems; regular and consistent time spent on the mat can boost immunity as it stimulates your lymphatic system; the rapid flow between postures will get your heart racing, enhancing cardio-respiratory fitness; and all those twisting postures will massage your digestive organs, which ultimately promotes healthy bowel movements – bonus!

YOGA AND SPORT

It's no surprise that professional footballers, tennis players and cricketers now include yoga in their training regime. They know the enormous benefits of the practice for increasing agility and balance while strengthening multidirectional joints – wrists, elbows, shoulders, knees, hips – reducing risk of injury. As yoga also teaches inner calm and focus, this strengthens a sportsman's resolve to win – and if he doesn't win, he's cool with it.

YOGA AND THE GYM

If you're a regular gym-goer, taking up yoga will make you stronger. The movement patterns of yoga equalise the flexibility between opposing muscles, which in turn increases your range of motion when lifting weights. This results in increased strength.

Yoga also improves your neuromuscular communication. This means increased balance and stability, which improves your form on the gym floor. And if you hit the gym regularly, you'll understand how important recovery time is. This is where yoga assists, as it decreases inflammation.

If you're not a gym guy, we do recommend you complement your practice with some strength training. As yoga focuses mostly on pushing actions, without much pulling, there's the potential for muscular imbalances. This can be avoided by targeting your back, posterior shoulder muscles and biceps with pull-ups, rows and bicep curls.

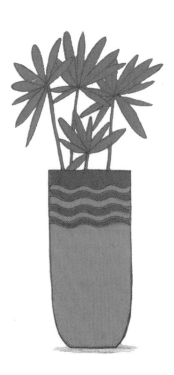

BREATHE

Your whole life happens between your first and last breath.

Just take a moment and think about that, while you breathe in – and out.
   Are you a shallow breather, only breathing into the upper respiratory tract? Are you a deep breather, inhaling into the lower depths of your lungs? Take a few moments to observe your breath and your body's relationship to it.
   If, like a lot of guys, you breathe rapid, shallow breaths, it could be that you're anxious or stressed, which can lead to insomnia and even sleep apnoea.
   When you're in nature – by the sea or in a forest – your body demands that you take in deep, wholesome breaths. Your diaphragm contracts and moves downwards, causing your lungs to expand, drawing in wholesome fresh air. You feel energised, awake, alert and connected. Now that is breathing.
   Yoga teaches you how to truly breathe. Without breath, there is no yoga. Breath is the most fundamental aspect of the practice. It roots us in our body. It connects body and mind.

In Sanskrit, the breath-work practice is called 'pranayama'.

Prana = Vital Energy. Ayama = Expansion.

Prana is the universal life force from which all energies stem. It's what allows us to experience life. It exists not just in our body, but all around us. It is the elements. It's both measurable and immeasurable. It's everywhere and nowhere and in all the places in between. Modern science has helped validate this concept of prana. Matter and energy are interchangeable as shown by the famous equation $E=MC^2$. In other words, the Universe is created by energy and that includes humans. More recent findings in quantum physics such as the string theory and Higgs field only reinforce the concept of prana. And prana rides on our breath. Now that's a concept to take your breath away!
   Pranayama is the practice of conscious breathing to expand prana within our body, in order to increase vitality and focus, to detoxify, and to calm the mind and nervous system. Pranayama enables us to explore the ways we can affect our breath, to change and regulate it, and thereby helps us to regulate our bodies too.
   There are many different pranayama techniques that we can apply to explore our breath and how breath affects us, for example 'ujjayi' (pronounced oo-jai-ee, meaning victorious breath), which is key when practising the postures, building heat in your body while encouraging calm and equanimity. Rather than breathing in through your nose and out through your mouth, like you do when playing sport or at the gym, ujjayi breath requires you to breathe in and out through your nose, with the length of the inhale matching the exhale. At the same time, it involves slightly constricting at the back of your throat, to create a sound reminiscent of ocean waves, or of Darth Vader! This technique allows you to stabilise your breath, even when the postures are challenging, and thereby stabilise your mind. But of course you're not expected to master this practice straight away. As a beginner you'll be taking it one breath at a time – and the rest will flow.

Nate's story

Imagine living your life from inside a shower, with a foggy piece of glass between you and other people. This is what it was like for Nate, before he found yoga. He wanted to connect with life but he just couldn't remember how. He had come to view the world through that murky glass curtain of depression. When did it start? He didn't know. Self-hatred, doubt and worry. They had all built, so slowly, over so long, that it was hard to pinpoint when it all began.

But things were definitely getting worse. And he was only 25. He was working four jobs at once, and hadn't taken a day off in months. It was long hours too, backstage in theatre, doing the same physical movements every day. Also, Nate talked to himself like shit. Any monkey could do this, his mind would tell him. What are you doing with your life?

Everything had become so vague and dark. He wasn't sure he even cared. Until he had an anxiety attack, and then all hell broke loose inside him. Nate had gone out the night before and woken up early for a job interview. He couldn't breathe and had no idea what was going on. Wheezing, shaking, frightened: it was like his nerves had taken steroids.

Nate stayed this way for five whole days. When he confided in one of his mates, they suggested he try yoga. After all, the studio was just around the corner from the theatre. There wasn't much to lose. So Nate went to a class – a turning point – and was hooked. Within a week he knew he had found gold. He'd go to work after class and practise, simply inspired to play and learn.

He loved the challenge of the postures, the concentration required and the heat that built inside his body. Yes, his ego came out like a storming monster sometimes, but he also learned to keep it in check, as his teacher drifted past him whispering 'easy tiger, keep breathing'.

In the yoga studio, Nate also picked up practical tools for his anxiety: breathing techniques, chants, but also simply things the teacher said (like 'fear is just excitement without the breath' – that one has stayed with him ever since). It sounds so simple to just focus on breathing, and yet this practice changed Nate's life. Experimenting with breath, exploring it and using it to access altered states of being; all of this has helped him with his anxiety more than anything else.

These days, Nate knows when he's becoming anxious as he's learned to observe his breath. And at the same time, he knows how to use his breath to calm his nervous system. As Nate continues to work on himself, he's now more attuned emotionally. Nate was the kind of guy who didn't cry, determined not to be like his father, a man he'd mocked many times for shedding tears at schmaltzy TV ads. But where does bottling it all up get you? Anxiety is usually a reaction to a trauma, after all, or a defence against deep feeling. It took a while – a couple of years, in fact – but at last he's letting go.

Everything Nate has been battling against his whole life – he's finally willing to let it in. Now he's the guy crying at the TV. What's more, it actually feels … good.

MEDITATE

Beyond the busyness of your mind there is a field of silence. An emptiness which is full. A stillness, which is dynamic.

How do you get there? You meditate.

But first, let's clarify something. Meditation is not something you do. It's more like the practice of not doing anything. It's something that happens to you, born out of the discipline of being still.

Meditation is about experiencing yourself as separate from your thoughts. Anxiousness, self-doubt, social conditioning, fear – these things begin to fall away, as do all your limiting beliefs about what it means to be a man.

Meditation is the deepening of your awareness of the silence within. The more access you have to that field of silence, the more access you have to your higher self, to nature's intelligence and universal consciousness.

If you've not yet experienced it, then just for now, you'll have to trust us: connecting to such stillness and silence is quite incredible. In this space, discord dissolves, pain heals and creativity arises. You tap into a field of high potentiality and self-discovery.

We know this might sound 'out there' but honestly, these are the facts. Contemporary research and neuroscience validates what the ancient yoga practitioners (yogis) knew: meditation not only heightens our sense of awareness but also improves our ability to focus, process information, reduce stress and tension, and increase emotional stability. Let's look at those benefits in more detail.

LESS ANXIETY

Daily meditation decreases activity in the 'monkey mind'. This is where your mind wanders from thought to thought in an anxious and restless way; thoughts about the past, the future, him, her, them…. This mind-wandering is typically associated with negative emotions. With regular practice, you can create new synaptic pathways in your brain that lead to a more positive relationship to yourself, addressing the source of your anxiety.

IMPROVED FOCUS

The practice of meditation focuses your mind. The more you meditate, the more your ability to sustain attention will improve when you're not meditating. It's like the way muscles strengthen as a result of regular exercise, and are then stronger for all activities.

Sharpening your focus will increase your mental clarity, give you more positive energy and enable you to disengage from negative thoughts faster.

INCREASED CREATIVITY

Meditation stimulates the neocortex, which is 76 per cent of the grey matter in your brain – the part of your brain associated with creativity, envisioning, problem solving and innovation. It is also the central hub for empathy, sensory perception, language, expression and motor commands.

Not only does meditation keep your creativity flowing, it also has the power to reduce the reactivity of your reptilian brain, the 'fight or flight' part of your brain that suppresses creativity.

THE POWER OF OM

In Sanskrit, a mantra is a sacred word or sound that is repeatedly chanted to help us to unhook from both our senses and our mind.

Man = heart. Tra = expansion.

It is said the power of mantra lies within your heart. More specifically, the rhythmic patterns of chanting change the electrical information that the heart generates and sends to the limbic region of the brain, deactivating negative thoughts and emotions. The powerful effects of this practice can lead you into a state of bliss, connection and transcendence.

The mantra 'Om', pronounced Aum, symbolically represents Birth, Life and Death. It originates from one of the oldest oral traditions, known as the Vedics. According to ancient Hindu scripture, Om is the cosmic sound that initiated the creation of the Universe. And likewise, cosmologists understand that the cosmic microwave background radiation from the Big Bang is the sound Om. So, when you chant Om you are tuning into the sound of the Universe and acknowledging your connection to it.

This sacred experience is amplified when humans chant together. We know first hand the power of 50 people reverberating the sound OM. A supernatural phenomenon happens. It's where biological systems become synchronised. The electrical signals of the heart go beyond your skin. We start to feel each other's electromagnetic fields. We vibrate as one. This interconnection between individuals is like a shoal of fish or a flock of birds in collective harmony. It is really and truly incredible.

So, now you know why we chant Om at the beginning and end of a yoga class. Because it opens your heart and centres you, connecting you to yourself, your fellow man and the Universe. Let's give it a go.

HOW TO CHANT OM

The sound Om is actually three syllables – and pronounced AWE-OOOH-MMMM. To access the power of this mantra, it is chanted as a deep, protracted vibration. This means accessing the lower register of your voice while maintaining a strong, upright posture. So, let's give it a go.

Sit with your spine tall, shoulders back and heart open.

To centre yourself, take three slow, deep breaths.

On the third exhalation begin to chant AUM.

Each syllable of the mantra will create a vibration within three different parts of your body.

AWE: The sound originates at your solar plexus, vibrating deep within your belly, moving up into your chest cavity.

OOOH: The vibration gradually rises into your throat.

MMMM: As your lips close, the vibration is felt in your mouth and inside your head as a prolonged hum.

Once the breath and sound fades, allow yourself a moment to pause. Repeat two more times.

Now that you've tuned into the power of OM, you're ready to start your practice.

LET'S GET STARTED

One of the great advantages of yoga is that you can literally do it anywhere. At home, in the park, on the beach, in a studio – just as long as you have a flat surface and your trusted yoga mat. We recommend you invest in the best quality one you can afford. It'll last you years and you can take it everywhere.

MAKING TIME FOR YOUR PRACTICE
Setting a routine will help create the time and space you need for developing your practice. In the same way you schedule work meetings or catch-ups with your mates, make an appointment with your mat and let everyone in your household know: this is your time for yoga.

WHAT TO WEAR
Let's be clear, you do not have to wear Lycra to do yoga. But we do suggest form-fitted, comfortable kit that allows you to move freely. Baggy clothes are not ideal; they interrupt your yoga flow and it's easy to get lost in them. As for socks, please, take them off. Yoga is a barefoot practice.

EXTRA BITS
Props, like yoga bricks, straps and bolsters, are handy additions to assist your yoga practice. They help raise you, support you and ease you into the various poses. As a beginner, your essential props should include:

A yoga brick, or two (you could also use a stack of hardback books)
A yoga strap (or a belt)
A bolster (or rolled-up blanket).

SET YOUR INTENTION
It's always good to bring a positive intention to the yoga mat as a meaningful way to focus your mind throughout your practice. It gives you purpose, motivation and inspiration. Perhaps there's something you wish to let go of, or something you want to activate. You may want to dedicate your practice to someone in your life who needs some good vibes sent their way. Or maybe your intention is simply not to fall over! Setting intentions on the mat allows your yoga practice to become a powerful tool for creating change, and not only in the physical sense.

WHEN YOU SHOULDN'T DO YOGA
Like with sport and gym work, if you're feeling unwell or if you've just recovered from an injury, it's advisable not to exercise – and this includes yoga. If you're on medication and/or have a chronic condition, you must have permission from your doctor before getting on the mat.

It's important to listen to your body as only you really know what's going on inside of you. Pay attention to any indicators of potential ill health. Breathlessness, light-headedness, heart palpitations and pain are all reasons to stop. Consult your GP before resuming practice again.

HOW TO APPROACH THE BREATH PRACTICES
Before diving into the postures, we recommend having a go at some of the breath practices first – after all, breath is the foundation of yoga. You will use your breath to deepen into the postures, to maintain your focus and support your practice. As we're not used to applying our breath as a tool, this is a really important skill to understand and develop.

The five different breath techniques in this book are designed for you to explore and have fun with. So try them all out and apply them to your yoga practice, and also in life.

HOW TO APPROACH THE POSTURES

As a beginner, you may find all of these postures (asanas) overwhelming. So where do you start? We suggest working through a few at a time from each category. We've grouped them into four clear sections: Seated Asanas, Standing Asanas, Inversions and Floor Asanas. Throughout we'll give you nudges, ideas on how to get the posture right, adaptations and 'warrior points' – because we're all warriors.

This book is both a guide and a reference source. Every posture is broken down and explained so that you'll have a full understanding of its purpose and how to do it. You might find certain poses relatively easy, but when you try others you'll be like, whoah. That's normal. Some guys are naturally flexible in their hips, others aren't. Some guys have stronger legs which means they can hold standing postures longer. Everybody's body is different. That's why we've included instructions for modifying each pose to make it simpler, along with tips for taking it to the next level. So just do what's achievable for you.

Over time, you'll develop a true sense of what you're doing, giving you the confidence to join a yoga class. And whenever you need further understanding, instruction or refinement, you have it all here.

UNDERSTANDING BASIC SANSKRIT

Sanskrit is the language of yoga. Steeped in tradition, myth and legend, it originated over 5000 years ago and is used to describe the various postures and practices you'll find in this book. While you don't need to know the full meaning of each of these Sanskrit words it would be helpful to start developing a basic relationship with them. We've also given you the phonetic pronunciation so that you can have a go at saying them out loud too.

HOW TO APPROACH THE MEDITATIONS

Later in the book you'll be introduced to some simple yet powerful meditative techniques where you'll use breath, visualisation, movement, focus and mantra to access stillness of mind. Before you give them a try, it's important to let go of any misconceptions you may have about meditating, especially the idea that you can't do it. You may be surprised by how naturally you can connect to presence once you have the tools and understanding.

HOW TO APPROACH THE SEQUENCES

This is the fun bit, where we bring together everything you've learned. Breath, posture and meditation unite to become what we call a 'yoga journey'. We've created five journeys for you to choose from, each with a different intention. Depending on how you feel on any given day, choose a journey that supports you. What does your body need? Where's your head at? What's your heart telling you?

So when you're ready to take your yoga journey, simply follow the sequence of poses across the page. We encourage you to return to the journeys as frequently as possible as this will embed the patterns of movement into your body – and before you know it, you'll be experiencing the power of a regular yoga practice.

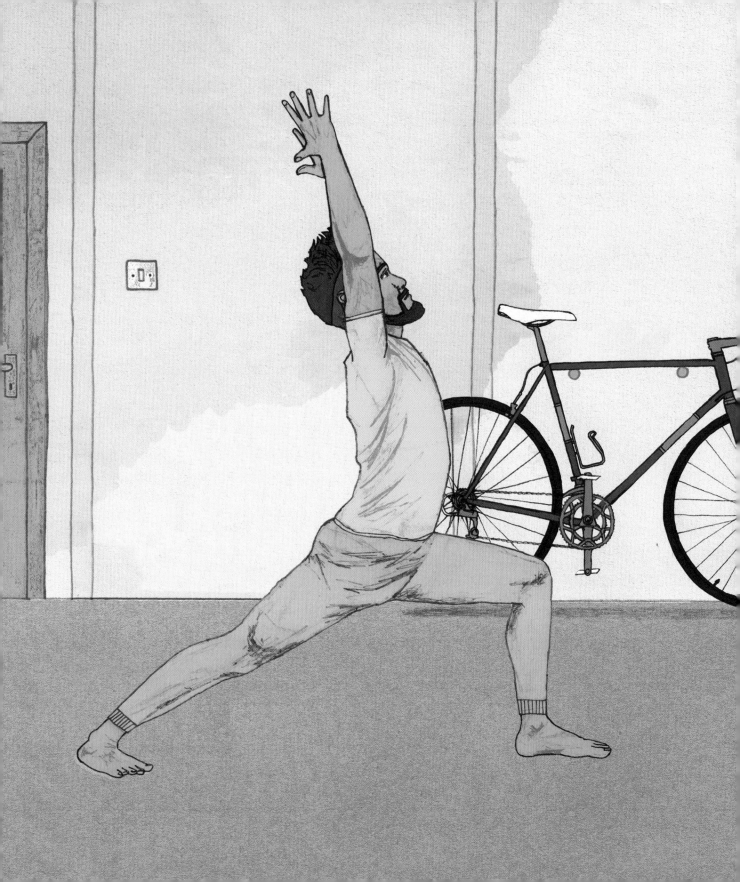

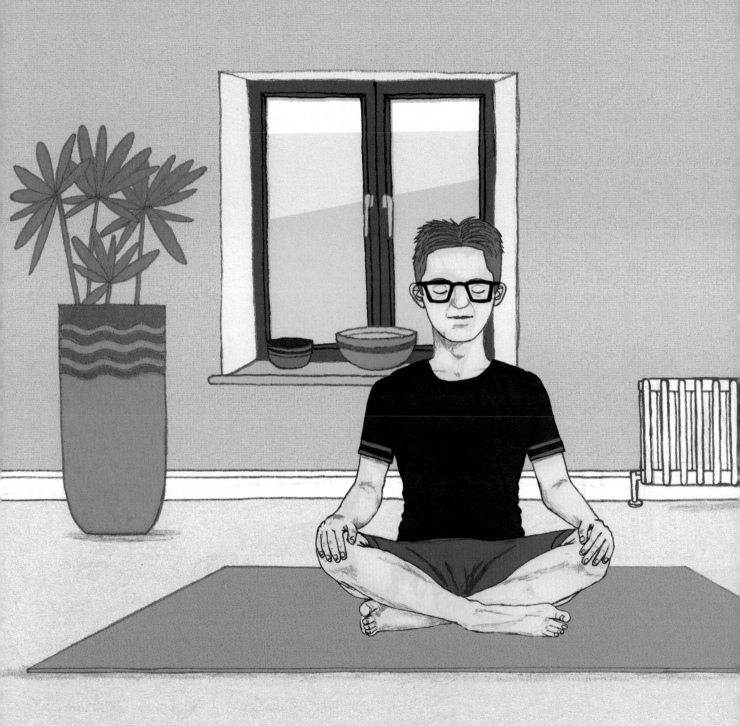

BREATH PRACTICES

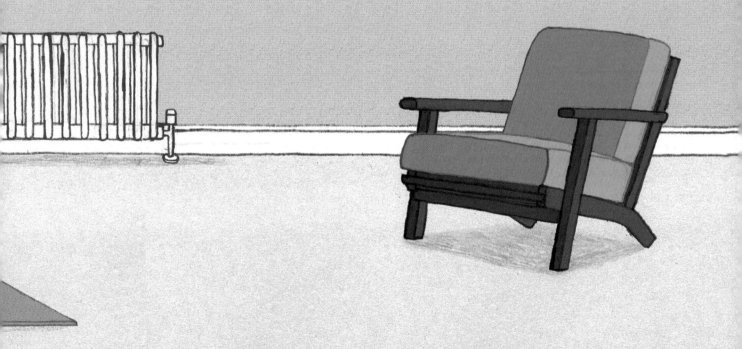

ALTERNATE NOSTRIL BREATHING
ANULOM VILOM

Anulom Vilom is a calming and stabilising meditative practice that you can use either before your asana flow or as a cool down at the end.

    As you control the flow of your breath through your left and right nostrils, you're activating both the left and right hemispheres of your brain.

    This level of concentration will centre your mind while creating peaceful, balanced energy.

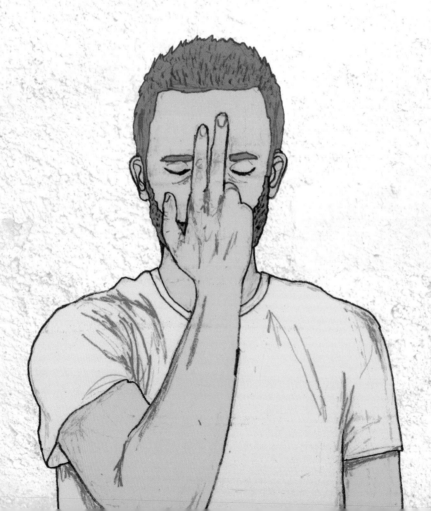

HOW TO DO IT

1 Begin in a seated position, such as Seated Pose or Hero Pose (see Seated Asanas, pp. 35–41). Make sure you're comfortable with your spine tall, shoulders rolled back and your chin parallel to the floor.

2 For this practice, you will use the thumb and ring finger of your right hand to open and close your left and right nostrils.

3 To start, bring your index and middle fingers together and place them between your eyebrows.

4 Close your eyes, bringing your awareness to your fingertips gently pressing against your Third Eye (see Glossary, pp. 154–5).

5 Close your right nostril with your thumb and inhale through your left nostril for four counts. Close your left nostril with your ring finger and hold your breath in for four counts.

6 Release your right nostril and exhale for four counts. Close your right nostril and hold your breath out for four counts.

7 Release your right nostril and inhale for four counts. Close your right nostril and hold your breath in for four counts.

8 Release your left nostril and exhale for four counts. That's one round completed.

9 Continue, for a minimum of five rounds, maintaining smooth, fluid breath.

YOGIC FOUR-PART BREATH

This foundational breath practice, also known as 'box breathing' or 'four square breathing', is a great introduction to pranayama. It will help you to get familiar with the flow of your breath, and the way your lungs, ribs, diaphragm and belly move while you breathe. Four-Part Breath teaches us how to equalise the four components of breath:

Inhalation (breathing in)
Inward retention (holding your breath in)
Exhalation (breathing out)
Outward retention (holding your breath out).

This practice helps reset your breath, enhance mental focus and quickly calm the nervous system, so it's a good one to use during stressful situations.

HOW TO DO IT

1 Begin in a seated position, such as Seated Pose or Hero Pose (see Seated Asanas, pp. 35–41).

2 Make sure you're comfortable, with your spine tall, shoulders rolled back and your chin parallel to the floor. Close your eyes.

3 Inhale through your nose as you count to four. Feel your navel gliding out, your diaphragm moving down, your lungs expanding. Visualise energy rising up from the base of your spine.

4 At the top of the inhalation, pause for four counts, holding the breath in. This is the inward retention.

5 Then exhale for four counts, softening your upper and lower chest and drawing your navel towards your spine. Visualise energy moving down your spine.

6 Pause for four counts, holding the breath out. This is the outward retention.

7 Then inhale again, continuing the Four-Part Breath, making sure that all parts are equal; the inhalation, exhalation and both the inward and outward retention.

8 Practise for at least three minutes for your first go, building it up over time.

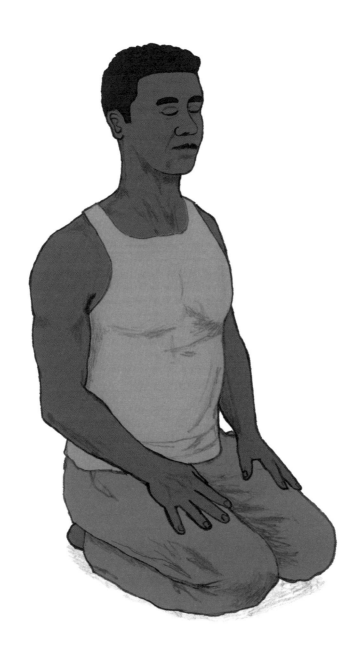

UJJAYI BREATH

Ujjayi, meaning 'victorious', refers to the partial contraction of the throat to control how you take in and release your breath. This technique is incorporated in many movement practices to help maintain a steady, rhythmic breath.

Ujjayi builds heat, enabling you to elongate deeper into postures, while encouraging calm and focus.

Tuning in to the audible sound of the ujjayi breath helps you to be more meditative during yoga practice.

Focusing on the ujjayi breath helps to anchor you in the present moment and diminish unhelpful distractions.

HOW TO DO IT

1   Begin in a seated position, such as Seated Pose or Hero Pose (see Seated Asanas, pp. 35–41). Make sure you're comfortable with your spine tall, shoulders rolled back and your chin parallel to the floor.

2   Close your eyes. Inhale through your mouth. Feel the breath pass through your windpipe and into your lungs.

3   Exhale through your mouth as you slightly contract the back of your throat to make a whispering noise like Darth Vader, or the sound of the ocean. You might also imagine you are fogging up a mirror with your breath.

4   Continue breathing in this way, contracting your throat on every exhalation. As you become comfortable, you can apply the same technique on the inhalation too.

5   Once you've mastered this technique for both inhalation and exhalation, close your mouth and breathe only through your nose. Now you're practising Ujjayi Breath.

6   Continue for three minutes, listening to the soothing sound of your breath.

7   Next time you practise the yoga postures, apply this breath technique to increase focus.

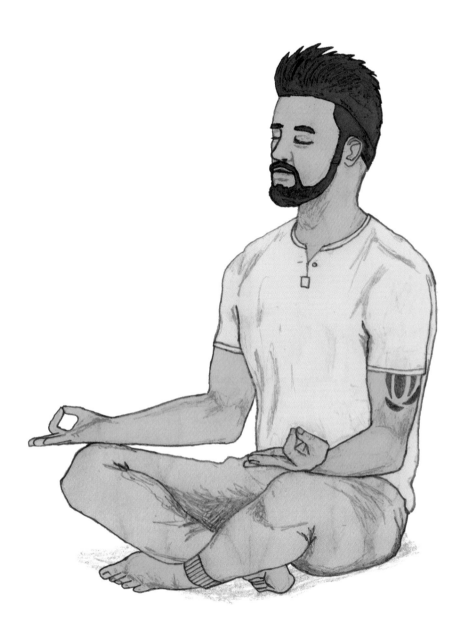

BREATH OF LIGHT
PRAKASHA

Prakasha means 'inner light' and that's certainly true of this breath practice, which really creates a feeling of lightness within your body. It builds a cooling energy that can calm fiery emotions such as frustration, impatience and anger. Breath of Light is a practice you can return to whenever you're feeling stressed or anxious. Just three minutes is enough to make a noticeable difference.

HOW TO DO IT

1 Begin in a seated position, such as Seated Pose or Hero Pose (see Seated Asanas, pp. 35–41). Make sure you're comfortable with your spine tall, shoulders rolled back and your chin parallel to the floor.

2 Close your eyes, bringing your awareness to your Third Eye. You'll find it right between your eyebrows – think of it is as the intuition power point!

3 Inhale through your nose in seven short parts of breath to create one full inhalation.

4 With every inhalation, direct your breath to your Third Eye while visualising golden light surrounding and permeating your body. It's not easy at first, but relax, and it will come.

5 At the top of the seven-part inhalation, hold your breath in for a few moments, focusing at your Third Eye, before exhaling in one continuous breath through your nose.

6 Repeat for a minimum of three minutes, creating a feeling of expansion with every breath as you invite more and more light into your body.

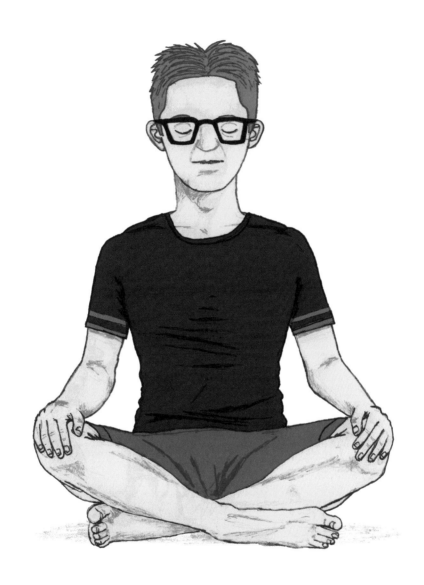

WARRIOR BREATH

This is a fierce and energising breath practice to connect you to your inner warrior.

Warrior Breath engages all of the muscles in your body to expand, release and transform energy while cultivating a grounded sensibility.

It uses your body's own resistance to strengthen, uplift and invigorate both physically and mentally. The next time you experience an energy dip, try some Warrior Breath practice – it'll wake you right up!

HOW TO DO IT

1 Begin standing with your legs wide, toes turned out and knees slightly bent. Tuck your pelvis by gently rolling your pubic bone towards your ribcage to flatten the curve of your lower back. Feel yourself grounded and stable.

2 Gaze straight ahead and extend your arms in front of you with a slight bend in your elbows, palms facing each other.

3 Inhale slowly in two parts through your nose: once, and then again. And with each small inhalation, arc your arms back, making fists with your hands.

4 Pause, expanding your chest and drawing your shoulder blades together.

5 Then exhale in two parts through your mouth as you move your arms in a two-part movement, returning to centre. By the end of the second exhale you should have palms facing each other.

6 Repeat five to 10 times with strong, deep breaths.

7 With every inhalation, think about contracting your back muscles as you pull through the resistance of your body.

8 With every exhalation, contract your chest, pushing through the resistance of your body.

9 Keep your face calm and relaxed – if you can!

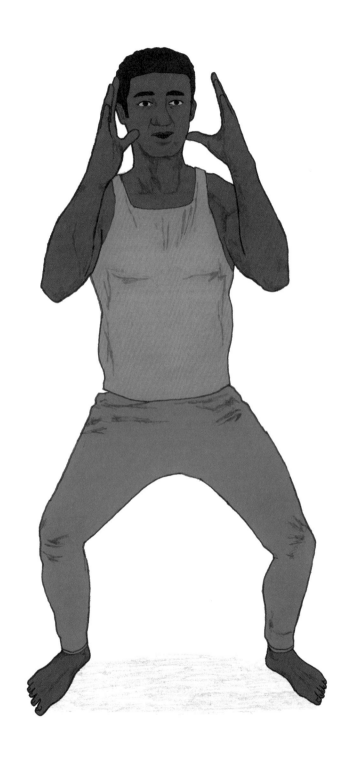

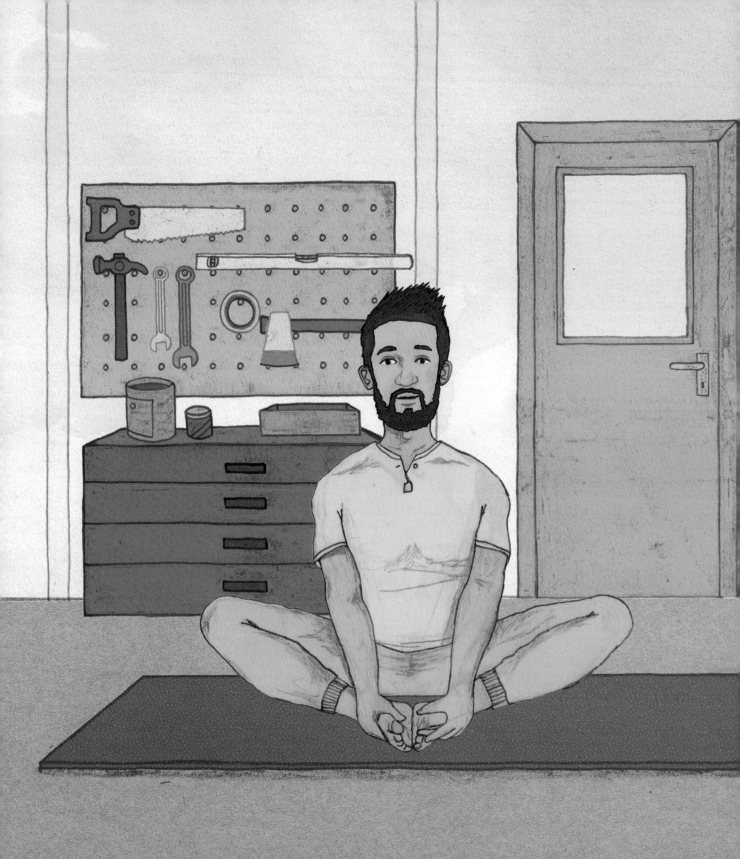

THE ASANAS

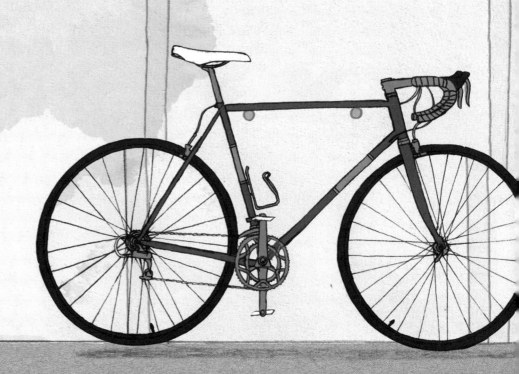

Caleb's story

In the first moments after my birth, I was separated from my biological mother. Put up for adoption, I spent five weeks as an infant in hospital before my adoptive parents came to take me home. Their love, security and nurture lessened the impact of this primal wound. But still, the pain of the separation was so profound it affected me on an emotional, psychological and cellular level.

I felt as though something was missing, deep inside. This sent me on a constant search for external validation, in relationships, career, fame – and more. Despite carving out a successful career as an Australian television presenter, I continued seeking, everywhere, for something – or someone – to fix me. I had no idea (yet) that true, grounded fulfilment comes from knowing that everything you need is within you.

I came to the UK aged 33, where I stumbled across spirituality. The true healing process had begun, igniting newfound creativity and purpose. Slowly, my ambition to be a famous TV presenter just … evaporated.

It wasn't that I went in search of yoga – more like yoga found me. Thanks to an acute inflammation of the connective tissue of the feet, I found myself barely able to walk, while simultaneously coming to terms with the disintegration of a long-term relationship. Taking a step forwards both physically and metaphorically was near impossible – and painful.

Many of my friends had mentioned yoga's ability to heal both body and mind, but I felt sceptical. I loved the gym and assumed that yoga was just gentle stretching, designed for those who were already able to touch their toes.

After trying every form of physical therapy, I finally took some time out for yoga. My first class, as well as the instructor, inspired and challenged me. After a few months, I could feel how getting on the mat was healing me from the inside out. Yoga was my physical rehab. And I developed the courage to finally walk away from my relationship.

So, with a broken heart and an open mind, I travelled to Rishikesh, a yogic hotspot in the foothills of the Indian Himalayas, where I picked the next available yoga teacher training: Sattva yoga. I had no idea about the practice, and limited understanding of anything beyond the physical postures. But as I immersed myself more and more, I felt my healing deepen. I witnessed myself in awe, as years of stuck energy released and all those old, limiting beliefs just disappeared. My early childhood, primal wound was at last really healing.

Best of all perhaps, I had now uncovered my purpose: to share this transformational practice with other men – the guys I saw everywhere who were cynical, stiff, stuck and full of pain. I want them to experience this freedom too. To feel and know the power of yoga.

SEATED ASANAS

Seated Poses are great for grounding you, centring you and bringing you into your body – which is why we typically practise these poses at the start and end of a class. And even though you're seated you could be crossed-legged, straight-legged, forward folding or twisting. Seated Poses focus more on flexibility than strength, which is great for an absolute beginner – especially as they can be adapted for any level.

EASY POSE

SUKHASANA

(SOO-KAHS-uh-nuh)

The original asana was simply this comfortable seated position that the ancient yogis took for meditation – which is how Easy Pose got its name. But these days, many guys find it far from easy sitting cross-legged on the floor, which is the reason why this foundational posture has so many benefits.

Easy Pose opens tight hips, while stretching your groin, inner thigh muscles, knees and ankles. It also strengthens your back and core. When practised properly with your spine strong, Sukhasana allows energy to move freely from the base of your spine to your crown (top of your head).

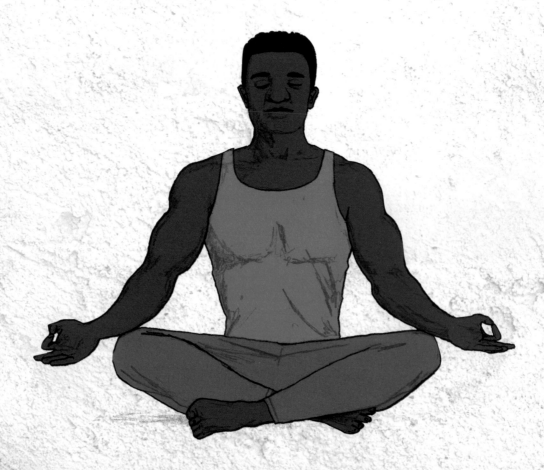

HOW TO DO IT

1 Sit tall on a yoga brick or rolled-up blanket with your legs extended in front of you.

2 Now cross your legs, with each foot resting beneath the opposite shin or knee.

3 Make sure that your hips are higher than your knees. If they're not, prop yourself up a little more.

4 Now, lengthen your spine, from the lumbar vertebrae to your crown. Imagine your head floating.

5 Roll your shoulders back and down to create an expansion in your chest.

6 Relax your arms, resting your hands on your knees, palms facing down or upward. If they face upward, you may like to try bringing the tips of your thumbs and index fingers together. Maintain a gentle forward gaze with your chin parallel to the floor, or close your eyes if you prefer.

7 Stay here for five slow, connected breaths, then change the cross of your legs for five more breaths.

○ WATCH YOUR FORM

Maintain your pelvis in a neutral position by ensuring your weight is evenly distributed across both your sitting bones.

Don't forget to change the cross of your legs. Holding the pose for the same amount of time on each side helps both hips to open.

○ HOW TO MODIFY IT

If you're finding it difficult to keep your back straight, try sitting up against a wall. You could also place a yoga brick between your back and the wall.

If you feel discomfort in your hips, knees or back, elevate your hips even higher. Go ahead and prop yourself up on an extra brick or cushion.

Warrior Point

When the base of our spine is grounded and solid, it sets the foundation for a healthy, strong and energised body.

HERO

VAJRASANA

(vahj-RAHS-uh-nuh)

Hero is a seated pose that stretches your
quadriceps and the tops of your feet, while
elongating your spine. This posture can help to
alleviate the kind of knee pain that is caused by
tight thigh muscles.

  You may find Hero Pose more accessible
than Easy Pose (with legs crossed, see
pp. 36–7) as it's easier to set your pelvis in
a neutral position, which takes the load off
your lower back. Vajrasana is a good pose for
meditating. You can sit for a while here without
developing backache.

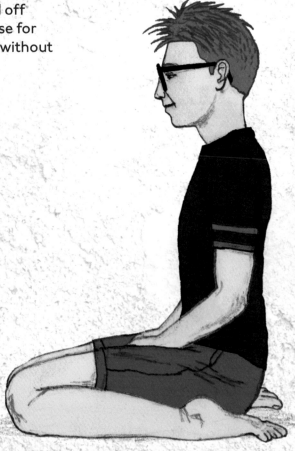

HOW TO DO IT

1 Start in a kneeling position with your knees together. Position your feet a little wider than hip distance apart with the tops of your feet face down.

2 Inhale through your nose. Then exhale through your nose as you lower your bottom to the mat. Depending on the size of your bum, you may need to move your feet accordingly.

3 Pull your navel inwards to activate your core.

4 Lengthen your spine, reaching the top of your head towards the sky.

5 Gently draw your shoulder blades together and down your spine.

6 Rest your hands on your thighs, either facing up or down.

7 Gently gaze forwards.

8 Stay here for five slow, deep breaths.

◯ WATCH YOUR FORM

Don't force it. Hero Pose can be an intense quad stretch, so take your time getting into the posture. And if you can't get your bottom all the way to the floor, sit on a cushion instead.

Make sure your weight is evenly distributed across both sitting bones, and also that the tops of both feet are pressing evenly into the floor.

◯ HOW TO MODIFY IT

To reduce the intensity of the stretch in your quadriceps and pressure on your knees, place a yoga brick or rolled-up blanket between your thighs to sit on.

You could also put padding under your ankles if they're uncomfortable in this posture.

↑ NEXT LEVEL

Once you've mastered Hero Pose, you may want to give Reclining Hero Pose a try. Lower on to one elbow at a time, then slowly lie back with your arms by your side.

Warrior Point

Being on your knees with a neutral spine enhances a meditative space, enabling you to go inwards to find stillness and peace.

BUTTERFLY

BADDHA KONASANA

(BAH-duh cone-AHS-uh-nuh)

Most men have tight hips, which can lead to lower back pain. Butterfly Pose is a simple, yet effective, starting point for opening up the entire hip area, including your groin, inner thighs, hip flexors and back.

This pose can also open us up to our internal feelings since our hips are considered to be the 'seat of our emotions'. Many men we have taught have described a release of deep emotions when practising hip openers like this one.

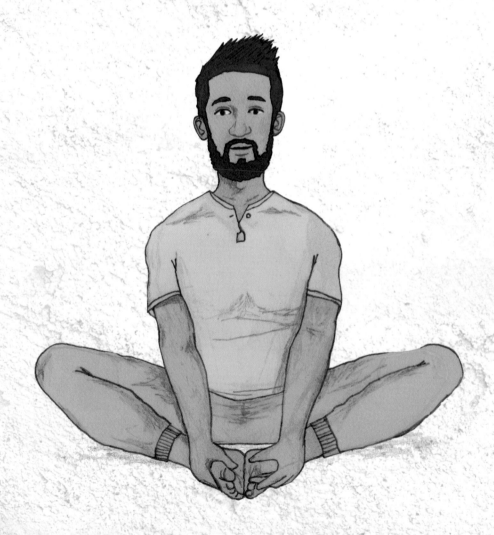

HOW TO DO IT

1 Start in a seated position with the soles of your feet together.

2 Feel your sitting bones pushing against the mat.

3 Grab on to your feet, ankles or shins (depending on how flexible you are) as you lengthen your spine.

4 Gently draw your shoulder blades together and down your spine.

5 Pull your navel inwards to activate your core.

6 Lightly gaze towards the floor.

7 Stay here for five slow, connected breaths.

○ WATCH YOUR FORM

Don't be tempted to push your knees towards the floor. Just focus on releasing the muscles of your inner thighs. You may not ever be able to flatten your knees to the floor – and this is okay. Your unique musculoskeletal structure will determine how deep you can take this pose. And any pose for that matter!

A common mistake is to hunch the back and drop the head down. Keep your spine lengthened by activating your core, drawing your shoulders back and visualising your head floating towards the sky (or ceiling).

○ HOW TO MODIFY IT

If you have lower back pain or sciatica, sit on a yoga brick or cushion so that your hips are higher than your knees. This will take the load off your lumbar spine.

Try experimenting with the placement of your feet. Position them further away from your groin to create a deeper stretch in your hamstrings. Bring them closer to your groin for a deeper stretch in your lower back.

↑ NEXT LEVEL

Try hinging forwards from the hips, maintaining a lengthened spine.

Warrior Point

Open hips = open heart.

CAT/COW

BITILASANA MARJARYASANA

(bee-tee-LAHS-uh-nuh mahr-jahr-ee-AHS-uh-nuh)

Cat/Cow is an essential part of any yoga warm-up, awakening the spine and preparing your body for the more intense postures to come. If you spend a lot of time sitting down, the spine can become compacted, resulting in a tight neck, lower back and hip flexors. Taking just 60 seconds out of your day to practise Cat/Cow will increase spinal flexibility by stretching your back muscles, neck and abdominals.

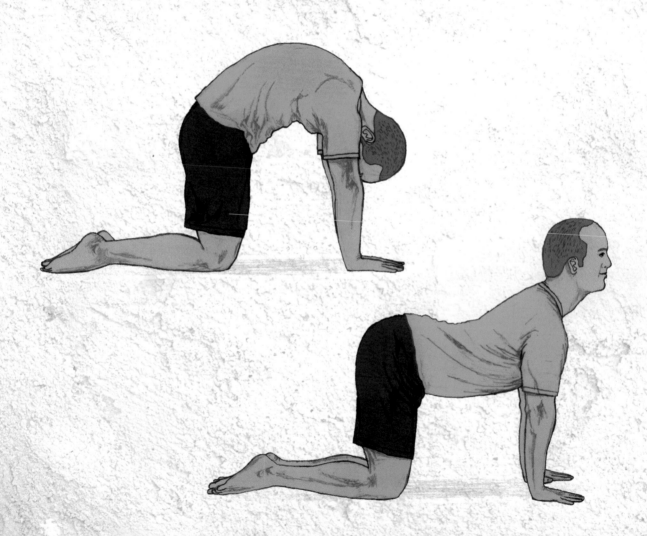

HOW TO DO IT

1 Start in tabletop position, i.e. on all fours, with shoulders over wrists and hips over knees. The spine should be neutral (neither arched nor concave) and parallel to the floor.

2 Next, bring your awareness to your tailbone – at the bottom of your spine. This part of your body should lead the movement into Cow Pose. As you inhale, move your tailbone towards the sky. Notice how your belly drops and your spine naturally arches. Lift your chest and your head, gazing forwards.

3 Now, as you exhale, you can flow straight to Cat Pose: scoop your tailbone under and draw your belly into the spine. Round your back and gently bring your chin towards your chest.

4 For another minute or so, continue flowing between the postures, inhaling as you move into Cow and exhaling into Cat.

○ WATCH YOUR FORM

When you move into Cow, be careful not to overextend your neck to avoid straining. Imagine there's an egg behind your head that you mustn't crack.

Your tailbone should lead the movement, with your neck and head following afterwards. As you inhale, the tailbone lifts; as you exhale, the tailbone tucks under.

○ HOW TO MODIFY IT

Are your knees hurting? Place a blanket under them for padding.

If your wrists hurt, support your weight with your fists. This can help strengthen the ligaments in the joint.

↑ NEXT LEVEL

Lift your right heel towards the sky, bringing your thigh parallel to the floor, knee at a right angle. Inhale to Cow, pressing your heel towards the sky. Exhale to Cat as you draw your knee to your chest.

Warrior Point

Practising Cat/Cow in synchrony with the breath encourages the mind-body connection. What is a mind-body connection? Really it just means listening to your body – and we don't mean with your ears!

SEATED TWIST

ARDHA MATSYENDRASANA

(ARD-uh MAHT-see-ehn-DRAHS-uh-nuh)

Seated Twist is an excellent movement for stimulating the muscles that support your spine, hips, shoulders and neck. Also, the rotational movement squeezes the abdominal area, which assists 'peristalsis', the involuntary muscle contractions that move food through your intestines. (Translation: this movement helps you poo! So if you have a slow, sluggish digestive system, Seated Twist is the ultimate detoxifier.)

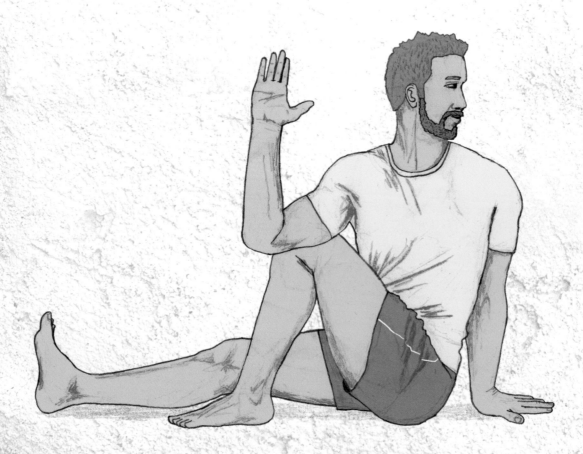

HOW TO DO IT

1 Start with your legs outstretched in front of you. Bend your left knee and place your left foot on the inside of your left thigh. Clasp your left knee with both hands.

2 Inhale and lengthen your spine, extending up through the crown of your head whilst pressing your sitting bones into the mat.

3 As you exhale, draw your navel towards your spine and start to twist towards the left. Think about making the rotation start in the centre and 'spiral' up your spine.

4 Take your left hand to the ground behind your butt and bring your right elbow on to the outside of your left knee. Gently press your elbow and knee against each other to ease yourself deeper into the twist. Gaze over your left shoulder.

5 Take three slow, deep breaths in this position. With every inhale, focus on elongating the spine more. With every exhale, focus on spiralling more deeply. Repeat on the left side.

○ WATCH YOUR FORM

Watch that your hips are parallel (rather than one lifted). Make sure you're grounding both sitting bones evenly to the mat before you rotate your spine.

Be careful not to lean forwards too much. It's important to sit tall to elongate your spine allowing for an effective spinal twist.

Be conscious not to initiate the twist from your neck. Rather, start twisting from your navel centre, spiralling up your spine, with your neck and head turning last.

○ HOW TO MODIFY IT

If your hips are tight, prop yourself on top of a yoga brick so that you can maintain a tall spine and reduce any strain in your hips, knees and back.

↑ NEXT LEVEL

For a deeper twist try positioning your left foot on the outside of your right thigh. And breathe.

Warrior Point

Spinal twists activate your solar plexus, located at your navel centre. Bringing this fiery chakra into balance helps cultivate willpower, self-worth and energy while eliminating self-doubt, insecurity and lethargy.

CHILD'S POSE

BALASANA

(bah-LAHS-uh-nuh)

Child's Pose is a position many of us adopted when we were little, and wanted to rest. Returning to this young place of nurture can be soothing, comforting and familiar, all of which makes it the perfect resting position within a yoga flow. It stretches the hips, quadriceps, ankles and back.

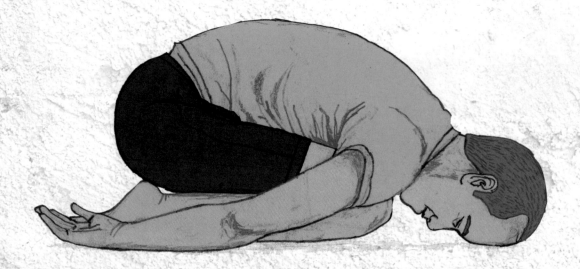

HOW TO DO IT

1 Start in tabletop position (see p. 43) on your hands and knees. Position your knees slightly wider than your hips, with your big toes touching.

2 Take an inhale, then as you exhale, sit back on your heels.

3 Next, walk your hands forwards a little. Inhale and extend.

4 Exhale as you sink your torso between your thighs, sinking your chest towards the floor. Rest your forehead on your mat as you soften and relax your lower back.

5 If it feels comfortable here then close your eyes and stay a while. Try walking your fingers further towards the front of your mat to lengthen through the sides of your back. Alternatively place your arms along the side of your body, towards your feet, with your palms facing up. As the front of your shoulders relax towards the floor, you will feel your upper back broaden; a nice, gentle stretch.

○ WATCH YOUR FORM

Ensure to maintain your neck in a neutral position. To alleviate any pressure on your neck, try resting your forehead on a cushion or yoga brick.

○ HOW TO MODIFY IT

If you can't reach your butt on your heels, place a cushion between the backs of your thighs and your calves for support.

↑ NEXT LEVEL

To make the pose more active, extend your arms in front of you, reaching your fingers towards the front of the mat.

To extend deeper into the pose, bring your knees wider apart, allowing your torso to sink towards the mat.

Warrior Point

Give yourself permission to slow everything down, to find comfort. Know that you're safe, nurtured and loved. No wonder toddlers often fall asleep in Child's Pose.

THREAD THE NEEDLE

PARSVA BALASANA

(PARS-va bah-LAHS-ah-nah)

Thread the Needle is a simple and accessible spinal twist that opens and stretches your shoulders, upper back and neck to help alleviate tension in these often tight areas.

    This pose is usually placed towards the beginning of a yoga flow, to warm up your body for the more challenging postures ahead.

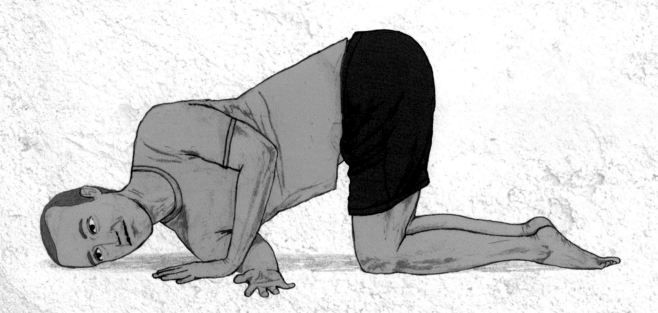

HOW TO DO IT

1 Start in tabletop position, on all fours, with shoulders over wrists and your hips over knees. Ensure your neck is neutral, with your gaze at the floor.

2 Inhale as you sweep your right arm towards the sky, following your hand with your gaze.

3 As you exhale, thread your right arm through the space between your left arm and knee. Bring your arm and shoulder down to the floor with your palm facing up. Rest your right cheek on the mat and gaze towards your right fingers.

4 Allow your chest to sink to the floor as you keep your hips lifted up and back.

5 Stay here for five slow, connected breaths. Or even longer if you want to. Then return to tabletop and repeat on your left side.

○ WATCH YOUR FORM

As Thread the Needle is quite a deep stretch it's important that you don't rush the movement. Practise with control, easing into the posture mindfully.

Are your hips lifted up and back? If your hips are positioned too far forwards this will place pressure on your neck rather than on your shoulders.

○ HOW TO MODIFY IT

If your knees hurt, place a folded blanket or towel under them as padding.

If you find the stretch in your shoulder too intense, rest your ear on a bolster or rolled-up blanket. This will raise your torso a little to reduce the pressure on your shoulder.

↑ NEXT LEVEL

For a deeper shoulder stretch, wrap your left arm around your lower back and rest the back of your hand on your right hip.

Warrior Point

Free your spine and the rest will follow. Keeping your spine healthy and supple is crucial for avoiding back issues and pain, and for ageing like a warrior!

STAFF

DANDASANA

(dahn-DAHS-uh-nuh)

This posture teaches foundational alignment for all seated postures, stretching your lower back, hamstrings and calves. Staff Pose is also a great spinal strengthening posture, activating the muscles in both your upper and lower back.

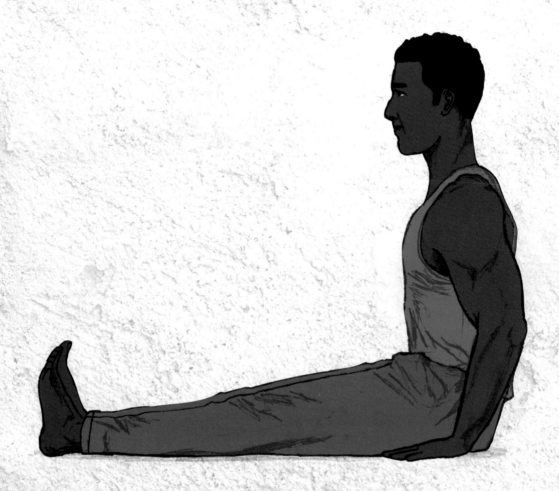

HOW TO DO IT

1 Sit with your legs extended in front of you and your weight evenly distributed across both sitting bones.

2 Engage your quadriceps and flex your feet so your toes are pointing towards your knees.

3 Place your hands on the floor beside your hips and roll your shoulders back and down, moving them away from your ears.

4 Inhale as you press into the floor and elongate your spine. You should feel a lengthening from the base of your spine all the way to the top of your head.

5 Gently gaze forwards.

6 Stay here for five slow, connected breaths.

○ WATCH YOUR FORM

Are you hunching over? This means you're not fully engaging your upper back muscles. Draw your navel in, roll up through your spine and draw your shoulder blades together.

Another common mistake is 'lazy legs'. Keep your quadriceps fully engaged as this helps to release the hamstrings.

○ HOW TO MODIFY IT

If you suffer from lower back pain, tightness or sciatica, try propping yourself up on a folded blanket or cushion.

You could also try leaning against a wall for support, ensuring your lower back, shoulder blades and the back of your head are all in contact with the wall.

If you're using a cushion for support, you may also need to pop a yoga brick under each hand.

↑ NEXT LEVEL

For a deeper hamstring stretch, try hinging forwards from your hips, reaching your fingers towards your toes. As you do this, maintain a lengthened and neutral spine.

HEAD TO KNEE FORWARD BEND

JANU SIRSASANA

(JAH-noo sheer-SHAH-suh-nuh)

This beginner's pose is a deep stretch for tight hamstrings, along with lower back, hips and groin. Head to Knee Forward Bend is made more accessible as it stretches one leg at a time, which enables you to comfortably go deeper.

   With regular practice Janu Sirsasana will become one of your more relaxing and calming postures.

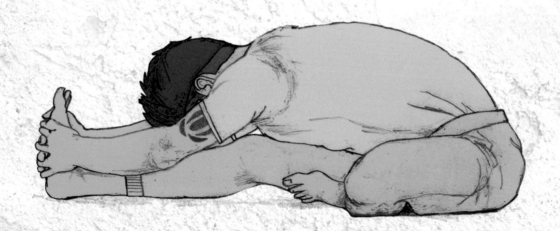

HOW TO DO IT

1. Sit with your legs extended in front of you, with your sitting bones grounded to the mat.

2. Bend your left knee, bringing the sole of your foot to your right inner thigh.

3. Flex your right foot, toes pointing towards your knee. Activate your quads and hamstrings, grounding your leg into the floor.

4. Square your torso over your right leg.

5. Inhale as you lengthen your spine.

6. Exhale and hinge forwards, reaching both hands towards your foot. What's most important here is to maintain a neutral spine. You don't want to hunch over, so reaching for your ankle or shin is perfectly okay.

7. Stay here for five deep, slow breaths, gazing forwards. On every inhale, lengthen your spine. On every exhale, deepen into the fold.

8. Repeat on the opposite side.

⭕ WATCH YOUR FORM

Don't round your back. The objective is to keep your chest lifted and spine lengthened.

Beware of sacrificing good form to reach your toes. Start with reaching for your shins, then your ankles, then your toes. It's all about progression.

⭕ HOW TO MODIFY IT

If you can't reach your foot, try using a yoga strap or belt hooked over the ball of your foot. This will enable you to gently pull yourself deeper into the fold.

If your hips are tight, prop yourself up on a yoga brick or rolled-up blanket.

↑ NEXT LEVEL

If reaching your foot while maintaining a strong elongated spine is easy for you, try interlocking your fingers over the ball of your foot.

Still too easy? Try both legs at the same time.

Warrior Point

Forward folds increase circulation to the pelvic and groin area, meaning increased libido and erectile function.

GARLAND

MALASANA

(mah-LAHS-uh-nuh)

This deep squat is a great posture to ease open those tight hips while also strengthening the feet and ankles.

   As little boys, we all spent hours in this posture, playing in sandpits or with toys. But as adults most guys have forgotten this primal position and will find it a real challenge.

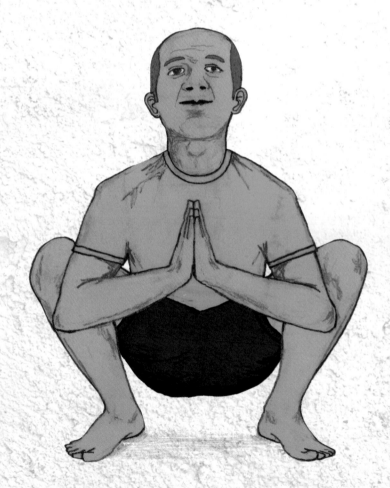

1 Start in a standing position with your feet mat-width apart, toes pointing out slightly.

2 Extend your arms out in front of you at shoulder height.

3 Maintain a neutral spine as you bend your knees and lower your butt, sending it backwards. Ensure your knees don't extend past your toes. If you can't see your toes, you're overloading your knee joints.

4 Once you're in the deep squat position, bring your upper arms to the inside of your thighs and bring your palms together into prayer position.

5 Lengthen your spine, lift your chest and draw your shoulder blades together.

6 Keep your head neutral and gently gaze upwards.

7 Stay here for five slow, deep breaths.

○ WATCH YOUR FORM

Are you on the balls of your feet? To get that deep hip stretch, you must sit back into your heels. If you need support, place a yoga brick, or two, under your butt.

If your upper back is rounded, lift your chest higher as this lengthens your spine.

○ HOW TO MODIFY IT

If you can't quite get your heels to the floor, you can roll up the end of your yoga mat and rest your heels there.

If you struggle with balancing, you can try this pose with your lower back pressing against a wall.

↑ NEXT LEVEL

Add in a spinal rotation by placing your left palm to the floor then sweep your right arm out to the right side and up towards the sky. Hold for five breaths as you gently gaze at your right hand. Exhale to release your right hand to the floor. Repeat on the opposite side.

Warrior Point

This posture is the ultimate eliminator! By stimulating and relaxing digestive organs, Malasana will help you release the poo.

BOAT

NAVASANA

(nah-VAHS-uh-nuh)

Here's a challenging abdominal strengthening posture that requires stamina, focus and commitment. Having strong abdominals will help you to master numerous balancing poses.

Boat Pose also strengthens your hip flexors, legs, lower back, upper back and shoulders.

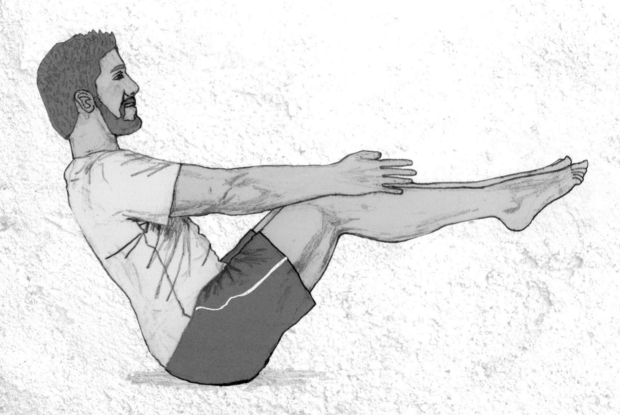

HOW TO DO IT

1 Start seated on your mat with legs bent and your feet on the floor – feet, knees and hips in alignment.

2 Grab the back of your thighs with your hands.

3 While maintaining a neutral spine, shift your weight back so you are balancing on your tailbone. Now slowly lift your feet off the floor, bringing your shinbones parallel to the floor.

4 Engage your core as you keep your spine lengthened.

5 Lift your chest as you squeeze your shoulder blades together, moving them down your spine.

6 Now release your hands and extend your arms forwards at shoulder height, with palms facing inwards.

7 Gently gaze forwards and slightly up.

8 Stay here for five slow, deep breaths.

9 Exhale to release your feet back to the floor.

○ WATCH YOUR FORM

Are you rounding your back? The objective is to ensure deep core engagement as this sets up your lower spine to support your entire back. And remember to squeeze your shoulder blades together to keep your chest lifted.

○ HOW TO MODIFY IT

If reaching your arms forwards is too challenging for you, then keep hold of the backs of your thighs. For more support you could place your hands on the floor behind you with fingers facing towards your hips.

↑ NEXT LEVEL

To further activate your inner thighs and hip flexors, place a yoga brick between your thighs and squeeze. For full Boat Pose, straighten your legs to a 45-degree angle while focusing on keeping your spine lengthened and chest lifted. The aim is to create a V-shape with your legs and torso. If you need some help straightening your legs, try wrapping a yoga strap or belt around the soles of both feet, keeping your feet flexed. Remember though, it's not worth compromising your straight spine in order to straighten your legs.

Warrior Point

Cultivate mental focus and determination with Boat Pose as these qualities will help you navigate through life's stormy waters.

Max's story

A self-confessed lad's lad, 25-year-old Max is not your average yogi. He left school at 16 with the dream of becoming an actor and stuntman. He was already a keen gymnast, snowboarder, skateboarder and martial artist, but yoga? Though it was his mother's chosen form of exercise, Max wasn't interested at all, assuming that the classes would be full of middle-aged women without any real strength. Eventually, more to placate his mum than anything else, he agreed to try it. Just the once.

Max was hooked after that first class. He was amazed to find the studio filled with fit people doing handstands and one-legged squats; an equal mix of genders. The practice itself had been humbling, leaving him satisfyingly exhausted, in a puddle of his own sweat. Max returned to class every day for a month. He loved the arm balances and inversion poses (in which your head hangs lower than your heart), as well as the mental clarity and relaxation he felt afterwards, both in body and mind.

Still aged 16 and by now a fledgling yogi (a source of great amusement to his teenage mates), Max flew to Miami to do a martial arts-infused yoga teacher training: 200 hours intensive, in just 12 days. Yet he still lacked confidence, and ended up working in an English hotel for 18 months, focusing just on his own practice rather than teaching anyone else. Max realised he wanted more. So he returned to the States to do further training in other styles of yoga.

After that, Max felt ready to teach. With his developing maturity, he began to subtly influence his mates to give yoga a go. He also showed them that it's okay to talk about their feelings. He became the guy they could count on for guidance and sage advice.

On a lads' night out, Max fell from a roof and broke his neck. His skull was also fractured, his jaw and eye socket injured, his wrist and palms mangled and he had blood coming out of both ears. That night, after receiving brain surgery, Max's parents were told that, due to a serious bleed on either side of his brain, he may not survive the night.

But survive he did and, 47 days later, Max returned home. When a physiotherapist arrived to treat him, he assumed he had the wrong house. The healthy, mobile, lucid young man standing before him couldn't possibly be the patient he'd read about. Given the nature of Max's injuries, it seemed inexplicable, explained the physiotherapist.

Max's surgeon agreed that his recovery was quite extraordinary. The only explanation she could find was that, because of Max's daily yoga practice, his brain was highly oxygenated on a regular basis and quite exceptional at regeneration. All the breath-work and mindful movement that Max had done meant that he was able to bounce back from his accident in ways that others simply wouldn't have.

Yoga didn't just improve Max's life. It saved it.

STANDING ASANAS

Standing Poses will literally have you on your feet – or sometimes just one foot! They cultivate balance, stability and strength, helping you build a strong foundation for improved posture and everyday movement patterns. Although challenging, Standing Postures can be invigorating and stimulating as they train your spine to move in all directions.

MOUNTAIN

TADASANA

(tah-DAHS-uh-nuh)

While this standing pose may appear like a simple yoga posture, it's actually one of the most challenging when done correctly. It cultivates balance and body awareness and requires a sense of focus and overall calm. It might look like you aren't doing much but, if you are doing it well, it is an active pose that subtly engages lots of different muscles simultaneously.

This is the pose that all of the other standing poses are founded upon, targeting your lower legs, thighs, hips, back muscles and abdominals. When practised regularly, Mountain Pose helps to reduce back pain and relieve sciatica.

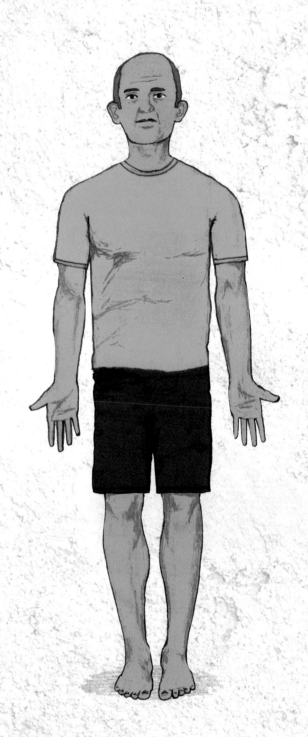

1. Stand up straight with your legs together or, if you feel wobbly, slightly apart. Take a moment to check your feet are parallel to one another, pointing directly ahead as any misalignment will affect the joints further up your legs (knees, hips and pelvis).

2. Lift and spread your toes apart before placing them back down on the mat. You should feel your weight evenly distributed across both of your feet. Rock gently back and forth, and side to side, until you come to rest naturally in your centre point.

3. Activate your thigh muscles, lightly squeezing them, feeling your kneecaps lift.

4. Pull your belly inwards a little. This will help to maintain the natural curvature of your spine and support your lower back.

5. Lift your shoulders towards your ears for a couple of seconds and then breathe out as you roll them back and downwards. You should notice your chest expanding slightly as you pull your shoulder blades together behind you.

6. Let your arms hang down by your sides, with palms facing forwards.

7. Keep your chin parallel to the floor and extend your neck as if someone is gently pulling the crown of your head up with a string.

8. Relax the jaw and eyes, softening your face and looking ahead with a relaxed, fuzzy gaze.

9. Stay in the position for five breaths, inhaling and exhaling through the nose.

○ HOW TO MODIFY IT

If you feel unstable in this position, move your feet so that they are hip-width apart.

Any knee issues? Keep the legs slightly bent to take pressure off your knee joints.

↑ NEXT LEVEL

Closing one or both eyes for a slow count of 10 is a great way to challenge your balance and focus, and helps you tune in more to bodily sensations.

Warrior Point

Experience yourself as the mountain; solid, grounded, expansive.

STANDING FORWARD FOLD

UTTANASANA

(ooh-tuhn-AHS-uh-nuh)

Standing Forward Fold is a powerful stretch to wake up your hamstrings – those long muscles at the backs of your thighs that get tight when you run, cycle, play football or sit for hours at a desk. When practised regularly Uttanasana also improves your spinal health, reduces back pain and eases tension from your neck.

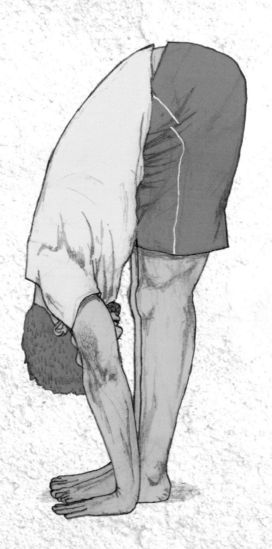

1 Start in Mountain Pose (see pp. 60–1) with your hands on your hips.

2 Breathe in and, as you exhale, bend forwards (think of hinging from the hips).

3 Fold your torso over your thighs as you reach your hands to the floor. If you can't touch the floor, that's okay. Just let your arms hang, maintaining a slight bend in your knees.

4 Activate the muscles down the front of your thighs (quadriceps) by squeezing them a little and drawing them up. This is really important because it helps your hamstrings to open.

5 Focus on placing your weight slightly forwards, just over the balls of your feet with your hips over your ankles.

6 Let your head hang and take five deep breaths. With every inhalation, slightly lift your torso. With every exhalation, release deeper into the fold.

7 To come up, bring your hands back on to your hips. As you inhale, activate your abdominals, lengthen your torso and rise up to where you began: Mountain Pose.

○ WATCH YOUR FORM

Don't make the mistake of flopping down into the fold and ending up with a curved spine. Instead, lengthen the backs of your legs and focus on keeping your back straight as you hinge forwards from the hips with control.

○ HOW TO MODIFY IT

Does the intensity of the stretch in the backs of your legs feel too much? Try bending your knees more. Alternatively (or in addition) place a block or stack of books under your hands for support. If that's still too much, rest your hands on the front of your shins instead.

↑ NEXT LEVEL

If you're very flexible in the hamstrings and this posture already feels easy, try grabbing your big toes then bending your elbows out to the side to deepen the stretch.

Warrior Point

Hanging your head lower than your heart calms the mind and soothes the nervous system.

CHAIR

UTKATASANA

(OOT-kuh-TAHS-uh-nuh)

Chair Pose is an energising standing
pose that gets the heart pumping by
using the largest muscles in the body;
your buttocks, thighs and upper back,
along with core and shoulders.

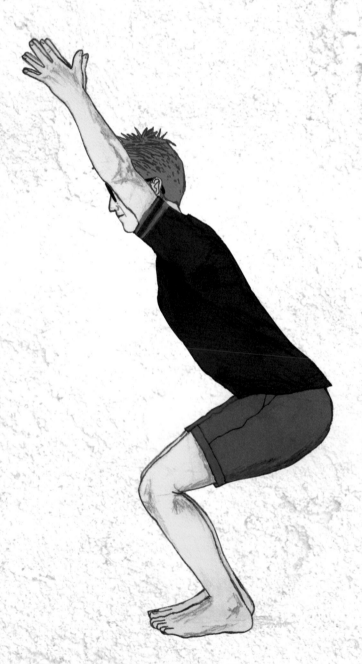

HOW TO DO IT

1 Begin in Mountain Pose (see pp. 60–1) with your feet parallel and hip-distance apart.

2 Hold your arms above your head with palms facing each other.

3 Shift your weight into your heels and begin to bend your knees, lowering your hips backwards until your thighs are almost parallel to the floor.

4 Ensure to keep your knees aligned with your toes as you activate your inner thighs.

5 With your butt low and chest lifted, aim to keep your arms in line with your ears.

6 Stay here for five slow, deep breaths while gazing forwards.

7 To release the posture, inhale as you straighten your legs. As you exhale, bring your arms to your side, returning to Mountain Pose.

○ WATCH YOUR FORM

If your feet are naturally pronated (roll inwards) or if they're supinated (roll outwards) pay particular attention to keeping them parallel, with your toes pointing forwards.

Ensure your knees are in line with your middle toe, not angled outwards or inwards. Can't see your toes? Your knees are too far forwards. Shift your weight into your heels and butt to correct your alignment.

Be conscious that you're not arching or rounding your back. Core engagement is really important here as it supports the lower back, so keep drawing your navel in towards your spine.

Avoid raising your shoulders up to your ears by drawing your shoulder blades down your spine.

○ HOW TO MODIFY IT

If you have difficulty balancing, try placing your feet shoulder-width apart.

If you're experiencing shoulder pain or tightness, holding your arms over your head may feel challenging. Try extending your arms forwards at shoulder height instead while drawing your shoulder blades together.

↑ NEXT LEVEL

Add a twist! Bring your hands into prayer position in front of your chest. With your feet parallel, twist to the right, bringing your left elbow on to the outside of your right knee. After five breaths, return to centre and repeat on the left side.

Warrior Point

In Sanskrit, Utkatasana means 'powerful pose'. Accessing your 'seat of power' strengthens your ability to fully support yourself in body, mind and spirit.

LOW LUNGE

ANJANEYASANA

(AHN-jah-nay-AHS-uh-nuh)

Low Lunge is an invigorating, deep stretch to relieve those tight hips and thighs. This is a posture to do often if you have a desk job or drive a lot, or if you run or cycle. It builds balance and stability, as well as opening the chest and shoulders.

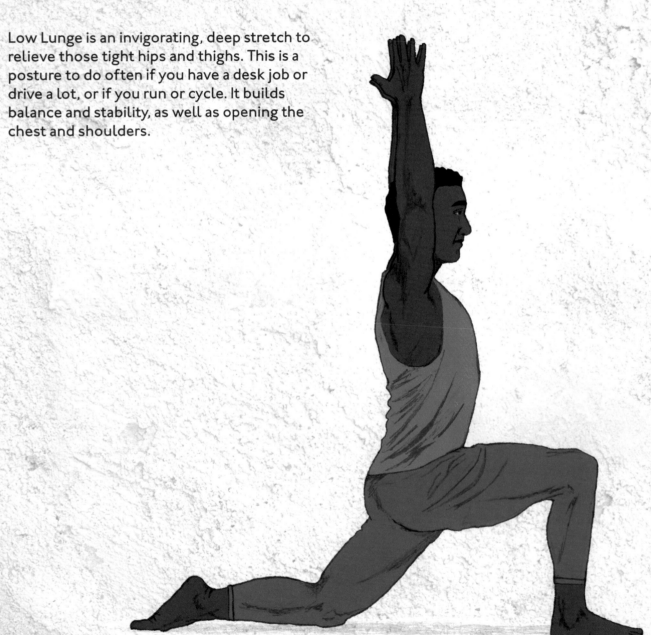

HOW TO DO IT

1 From a Forward Fold (see pp. 62–3), place both hands on to the floor and step your left foot to the back of your mat. Lower your left knee on to the mat and untuck your toes.

2 Inhale as you sweep your arms above your head, bringing them in line with your ears.

3 Draw your navel in towards your spine. This activates the deep core muscles.

4 Sink your hips forwards and downwards, deepening into the lunge.

5 To activate, draw your left knee forwards and your right ankle backwards, squeezing your left buttock.

6 Make your arms strong and active, extending towards the sky. At the same time, draw your shoulder blades down your spine to create space between your ears and shoulders.

7 If it feels comfortable, arch back a little into a slight backbend.

8 Stay here for five slow, deep breaths.

9 Exhale as you release your hands to the floor. Step your left foot forwards, then step your right foot back to repeat on the opposite side.

○ WATCH YOUR FORM

It's common to overextend into the lunge and push the knee too far forwards, placing strain on the joint. To avoid this, keep your shinbone perpendicular to the floor.

Always check the position of your back foot, which should be straight, with the top of your foot in contact with the mat.

○ HOW TO MODIFY IT

If your hip flexors and quadriceps are tight, keep the front knee at a 90-degree angle with the floor.

If it's painful to rest your back knee on the floor, put a cushion under it for support, or double your yoga mat to create padding.

If you're struggling with balance, try tucking your back toes under to create stability.

↑ NEXT LEVEL

To increase the stretch, shift your front foot forwards a few inches and sink your hips forwards and down. Be mindful not to overload your knee.

To add a deep thigh stretch, bend your back leg and take hold of your ankle with the hand on that same side. Slowly pull your heel towards your butt.

Warrior Point

Low Lunge is both grounding and expansive. Strong foundations will support you when reaching for your highest potential.

WARRIOR I
VIRABHADRASANA I
(veer-ah-bah-DRAHS-uh-nuh one)

Warrior I is no ordinary lunge. This foundational posture will test your stability, focus and body awareness. It's great for strengthening your thighs, calves and ankles while stretching your chest, shoulders, neck and groin.

HOW TO DO IT

1 From Mountain Pose (see pp. 60–1), step your right foot to the back of your mat, pivoting it into a 45-degree position and grounding your heel into the floor.

2 The heel of your left foot should be in line with the arch of your right foot. And your right foot should be fully connected to the mat.

3 Position your left knee over your left ankle so that your shin bone is perpendicular to the floor. Check that you can see your big toe. If you can't, reposition your knee.

4 Square your hips to the front of your mat by drawing your right hip forwards and left hip back.

5 Inhale as you sweep your arms towards the sky, gently lifting your chest to extend your spine.

6 Gaze slightly upwards while drawing your shoulder blades down your spine.

7 Hold for five slow, connected breaths.

8 Inhale as you step your right foot forwards to the front of the mat, then exhale as you lower your arms, returning to Mountain Pose. Repeat on the opposite side.

○ WATCH YOUR FORM

Avoid overloading the knee joint by ensuring that your front shinbone stays perpendicular to the floor.

Are your hips square to the front of the mat? Not sure? Place your hands on the bony bits of your hips and straighten them up so that both hips are equal distance to the front of the mat.

○ HOW TO MODIFY IT

Aligning your front heel with the arch of your back foot may feel like you're trying to balance on a tightrope. An easier option is to place your feet wider as if standing on railway tracks.

↑ NEXT LEVEL

For an added chest stretch try bringing your hands behind your lower back, interlocking your fingers. Draw your shoulder blades together while wrapping your triceps (backs of your upper arms) towards the back of the mat to expand your chest.

Warrior Point

With alignment and awareness you will awaken the warrior within.

WARRIOR II

VIRABHADRASANA II

(veer-ah-bah-DRAHS-uh-nuh two)

Warrior II is a fierce standing posture that enhances stamina, stability and concentration. It offers a powerful stretch for your legs, groin and chest, while also strengthening your legs, arms, shoulders and core.

This posture intensifies your focus and determination, which enables you to tap into your inner warrior.

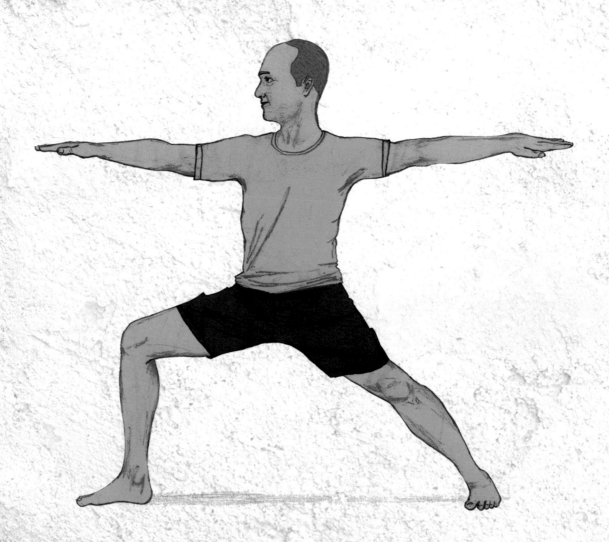

1 Begin in Warrior I (see pp. 68–9), ensuring your feet are positioned correctly with your right knee stacked over your right ankle.

2 Rotate your hips so that you're facing the side of your mat. Then extend your arms wide, reaching your right arm towards the front of the mat and your left arm towards the back. Keep your arms parallel to the floor with palms facing down.

3 Drop your shoulders away from your ears and expand your chest.

4 Turn your head towards the front of the mat and gaze over your right fingertips.

5 Stay here for five slow, deep breaths.

6 Exhale as you bring both hands to the floor, either side of your right foot. Step your left foot forwards then repeat on the opposite side.

WATCH YOUR FORM

Avoid overloading the knee joint by ensuring that your front shinbone stays perpendicular to the floor. If your knees collapses inwards, engage your adductors (inner thigh muscles) and re-align your knee with your middle toe.

Keep your triceps engaged, and the arms active with fingers stretched and pointed.

HOW TO MODIFY IT

If you have neck pain and find it uncomfortable turning your head towards the front of the mat, switch to a neutral position with your head and torso facing the same direction.

If you have a shoulder injury, or are feeling any pain in your shoulders, just bring your hands to your hips and focus on strongly engaging your legs.

↑ NEXT LEVEL

Activate your arm and shoulder muscles even more by turning your palms to face upwards, and externally rotating your arms. As you do this, you'll feel your triceps engage and chest expand. Now turn your palms to face downwards again while trying to maintain that external rotation of the shoulders and continuing to squeeze your triceps.

Warrior Point

The clue is in the name. Holding this posture with full engagement of all the required muscles is no easy feat. It'll get you strong, both mentally and physically.

WARRIOR III

VIRABHADRASANA III

(veer-ah-bah-DRAHS-uh-nuh three)

Sometimes known as Superman Pose or Flying Dragon, this posture not only requires power and stability but also a lightness of being as you float your back leg. It builds strength in the buttocks, legs, ankles, feet, shoulders and core. And because you stabilise yourself on one leg, Warrior III calls for acute mental focus, which does take some practice.

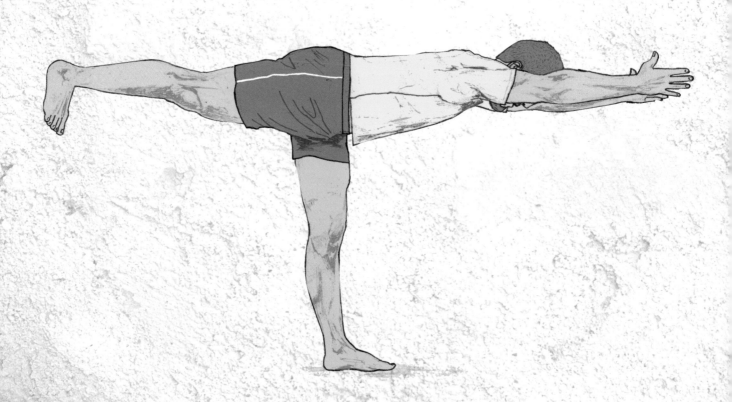

HOW TO DO IT

1 Begin in Warrior I (see pp. 68–9), with your left foot forwards, and right leg extended to the back of the mat.

2 With your hands on your hips, lean forwards and bring your weight into your left foot.

3 Pull your navel into your spine to engage your core as you float your right leg towards the sky.

4 Bring your torso forwards as you counterbalance, lifting and extending your right leg upwards. The objective is that your floating leg and torso will become parallel to the floor.

5 Keep your neck neutral and your head just as it would be if you were standing upright. Maintain a gentle gaze at the floor.

6 Fully extend your right leg while flexing your foot – toes pointing towards your knee.

7 Try to keep your hips level. It's normal for the left hip to tilt upwards, so use your core strength and try to keep your hips as square as possible.

8 When you feel stable enough, extend your arms forwards alongside your ears. Feel that dynamic energy moving from your back heel all the way to your crown – now you know why it's called 'Superman' posture!

9 Stay here for five slow, deep breaths.

10 Exhale as you re-bend the left knee and lower the right leg, returning to Warrior I.

○ WATCH YOUR FORM

Protect your knee joint on the standing leg by never locking it out or hyperextending your knee. Instead, maintain a very slight bend in your knee and engage the calf muscles for support.

To prevent your neck from straining upwards or hanging too low, focus your gaze on the floor, keeping your spine neutral.

Be conscious that your rear leg doesn't extend too high (this places increased pressure on your lower back).

○ HOW TO MODIFY IT

If this posture seems impossible for you, try holding the back of a sturdy chair. This will give you added stability as you float your back leg upwards and bring your torso parallel to the floor.

↑ NEXT LEVEL

Try playing around with arm positions. You can extend your arms forwards, in line with your ears. You can expand your arms out to the side like an aeroplane. Or, you can bring your hands together, in prayer position at your heart centre.

Warrior Point

The warrior takes flight with both strength and grace, two qualities essential for joyful self-mastery.

TREE

VRKSASANA

(vrik-SHAH-suh-nuh)

This is one of the simplest, and yet, most
challenging postures in yoga, requiring
balance, core strength and concentration.
Tree Pose strengthens and stabilises your
hips, legs, knees, ankles and feet, while
also stretching your inner thigh muscles
and groin.

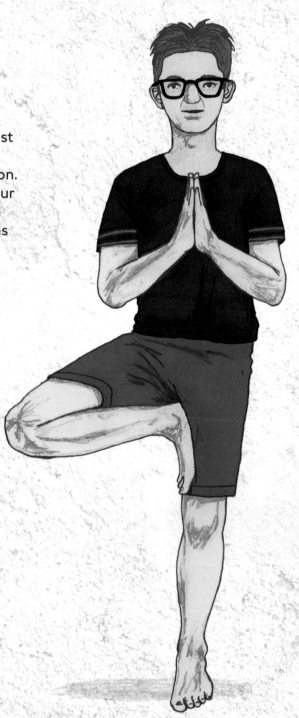

HOW TO DO IT

1 Begin in Mountain Pose (see pp. 60–1) with both feet firmly grounded.

2 Shift your weight on to your left foot. Keep the left leg straight but do not entirely lock out your knee – maintain a micro-bend instead.

3 Bring the sole of your right foot to the middle of the inside of your left leg, either below or above the knee. Press the foot against the leg and the leg against the foot, with equal pressure.

4 Keep your hips facing directly forwards, square to the front of the mat.

5 Bring your hands together at your heart as you gently gaze straight ahead.

6 Stay here for five slow, deep breaths.

7 Lower your right foot to the floor and repeat on the opposite side.

○ WATCH YOUR FORM

Ensure your hips remain in a neutral position by engaging your buttock muscles on the standing leg, as well as activating your core muscles.

Avoid placing the lifted foot directly on the knee of the standing leg as this puts too much pressure on the joint.

○ HOW TO MODIFY IT

If you're struggling to balance in this posture, practise against a wall, just until you get the hang of it.

Another beginner version is to place the lifted foot against the inside of your ankle (instead of thigh) and keep your toes on the floor.

↑ NEXT LEVEL

To challenge your balance further, lift your arms above your head in a V-shape.

Still too easy? Close your eyes to really stimulate your proprioceptive senses (those that tell you where your body is in space).

Warrior Point

This posture makes you Zen as a monk. Especially when you can perform it with both eyes closed, smiling.

TRIANGLE

UTTHITA TRIKONASANA

(oo-TEE-tah tree-koh-NAHS-uh-nuh)

This foundational posture is both lengthening and strengthening. It deeply stretches your hamstrings, groin and hips while activating your quadriceps, knees and ankles in order to open your chest and shoulders. Both balance and stability are essential to hold your body in this triangle shape.

1 Begin in Warrior II (see pp. 70–1) with your right foot forwards and arms parallel to the floor.

2 Inhale as you straighten your right leg. It's important not to lock out your knee but rather maintain a micro-bend as you engage your upper thighs.

3 Exhale, extending your right arm towards the front of the mat as you press your left hip towards the back of the mat.

4 Slowly lower your right hand to rest on your shin, ankle, or, if it feels comfortable, to the floor, just on the inside of your right foot.

5 Extend your left arm to the sky, keeping your left shoulder stacked over the right shoulder.

6 Gaze up to your left fingertips as you draw your shoulder blades together, opening the chest.

7 Keep your right quadriceps activated, maintaining that micro-bend in your knee.

8 Stay here for five slow, deep breaths.

9 When you're ready to come up, ensure your core is switched on. Inhale as you rise up and exhale as you re-bend your right knee, returning to Warrior II.

○ WATCH YOUR FORM

Correct foot alignment is key, so check your right heel is in line with the middle of your left foot.

If you're unable to reach your shin, that's okay. Just make sure you're not resting your hand directly on your knee joint.

○ HOW TO MODIFY IT

If tightness in your neck is restricting you from looking up at your fingertips, no worries. Just keep your head in a neutral position, gazing forwards instead.

You can also gaze down at the hand resting on your shin if that feels more comfortable.

↑ NEXT LEVEL

To further test your balance and core stability, try hovering your right hand over the floor. Don't forget to breathe!

Warrior Point

Triangle Pose is known for its strength and ability to support its load, just like the Pyramids of Giza. Think of this yoga posture as an engineering structure, perfectly balanced and solid.

EXTENDED SIDE ANGLE

UTTHITA PARSVAKONASANA

(oo-TEE-tah PARZH-vuh-ko-NAHS-uh-nuh)

This energy-boosting standing pose utilises all the muscles in your body, while lengthening through the entire side of your body, from your feet to your fingers. Extended Side Angle stretches and strengthens hamstrings, hips, groin and abdominals while opening your chest and shoulders.

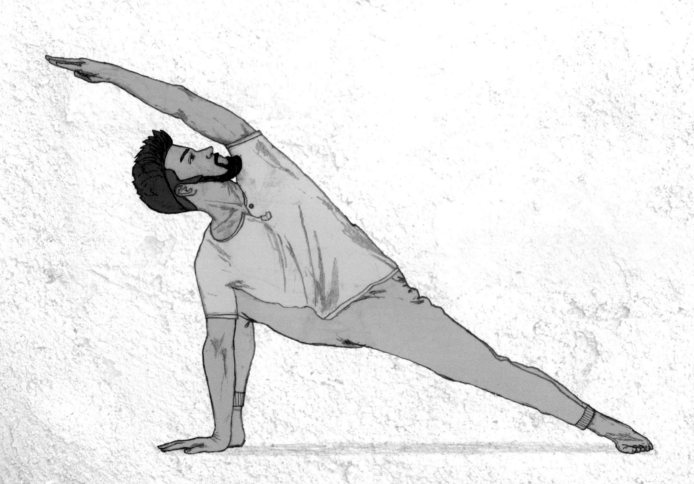

HOW TO DO IT

1 From Mountain Pose (see pp. 60–1), step your left foot to the back of your mat, pivoting it into a 45-degree position and grounding your heel into the floor.

2 The heel of your right foot should be in line with the arch of your left foot. And your left foot should be fully connected to the mat.

3 Position your right knee over your right ankle so that your shin bone is perpendicular to the floor. Check that you can see your big toe. If you can't, reposition your knee.

4 Turn to face the left side of your mat and extend your arms so they are parallel to the floor.

5 Bend your right knee, positioning it over your right ankle. Your thigh should be parallel to the floor. Reposition your feet if you need to.

6 Rest your right forearm on your thigh, with your palm facing the sky.

7 Inhale as you sweep your left arm up and over your head, extending all the way to your fingertips.

8 Rotate your torso, opening your chest towards the sky.

9 Gently gaze towards your left hand.

10 Stay here for five slow, connected breaths.

11 Inhale to bring your torso upright, arms parallel to the floor. Exhale and step your left foot to the front of your mat, returning to Mountain Pose. Repeat on the opposite side.

○ WATCH YOUR FORM
Watch out for overloading your front knee. It's important to maintain a 90-degree angle at your knee, with your knee stacked over your ankle.

Don't let the front knee collapse inwards. This is common if you have tight hips. To correct this, engage your adductors (inner thigh muscles) and line up your knee with your middle toe.

Is your back heel lifting off the floor? The aim is for the entire foot to be grounded to the mat. If you're struggling, practise with your foot positioned against a wall. By pressing your foot into the wall, you will feel more support.

○ HOW TO MODIFY IT
If you have shoulder pain and it feels uncomfortable to extend your arm over your head, try extending your arm perpendicularly to the floor instead.

If neck pain makes it difficult for you to gaze up to your hand, turn your gaze to the side or to the floor instead.

↑ NEXT LEVEL
For a deeper variation of Extended Side Angle, try bringing your lower hand to the floor, or to rest on a yoga brick. Make sure your chest doesn't drop to face the floor though. Keep rotating your torso so your chest opens to the sky.

Warrior Point
As you rotate your chest, and therefore your heart centre towards the sky, you're opening the channels to self-care. Welcome in the power of love.

REVERSE WARRIOR

VIPARITA VIRABHADRASANA

(VIP-uh-REE-tuh veer-ah-buh-DRAHS-uh-nuh)

Here's a deep side stretch for your torso that's done in a lunge position. As well as improving spinal flexibility, Reverse Warrior strengthens and stretches your hamstrings, quadriceps, groin, hips, shoulders and arms. In a class, you would typically flow to Reverse Warrior from Warrior II (see page xx) as part of a sequence to build energy and stamina.

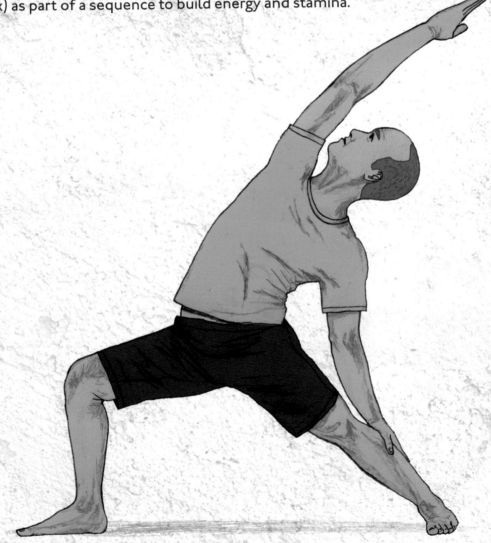

1 From Mountain Pose (see pp. 60–1), step your left foot to the back of your mat, pivoting it into a 45-degree position and grounding your heel into the floor.

2 The heel of your right foot should be in line with the arch of your left foot. And your left foot should be fully connected to the mat.

3 Position your right knee over your right ankle so that your shin bone is perpendicular to the floor. Check that you can see your big toe. If you can't, reposition your knee.

4 Turn to face the left side of your mat and extend your arms so they are parallel to the floor.

5 Bend your right knee, positioning it over your right ankle. Your thigh should be parallel to the floor. Reposition your feet if you need to. Feel familiar? That's because you're in Warrior II pose.

6 Now let's reverse your warrior! Turn your right palm to the sky. Inhale and sweep your right arm up and over your head.

7 Bring your left hand to rest gently on the back of your left thigh.

8 Maintain your right knee at a right angle. Keep your chest lifted and gaze at your right fingertips.

9 Stay here for five deep, slow breaths.

10 Each time you inhale, reach your right fingertips higher, lengthening the right side of your body. With every exhale, slide your left hand further down your left leg, deepening into the side bend.

11 Inhale to bring your torso upright, arms parallel to the floor. Exhale as you step your left foot to the front of your mat, returning to Mountain Pose. Repeat on the opposite side.

○ WATCH YOUR FORM

Ensure your front knee is at a 90-degree angle. As you lean back, the natural inclination is for your knee to move with you. The aim is to keep your knee stacked over your ankle so, once you've established the pose, check your knee is in alignment.

Also, don't allow your front knee to collapse inwards. This is common if you have tight hips. To correct this, engage your adductors (inner thigh muscles) and align your knee with your middle toe.

Beware of placing weight against your back thigh with your back hand. Use your core to stabilise yourself.

○ HOW TO MODIFY IT

If you have tight hips, try shortening your stance with the angle of your front knee slightly more than 90 degrees.

If you're feeling unstable, try placing the outer edge of your back foot against a wall. By pressing your foot into the wall, you will feel more support.

↑ NEXT LEVEL

For an added shoulder stretch, try wrapping your left arm around your back with your fingers reaching towards your inner right thigh.

Warrior Point

Standing poses help to cultivate poise and grace. We don't need to tell you why that's important, do we?

PYRAMID

PARSVOTTONASANA

(PARZH-voh-tahn-AHS-uh-nuh)

This pose simultaneously stretches hamstrings and shoulders while building balance and coordination. Pyramid Pose will also stretch and strengthen the entire spine, hip, knee and ankle joints as well as improve core strength.

Pyramid is an inversion pose, so you'll be hanging your head upside down, meaning more blood flow to your head. This can help with calming your mind and therefore reduces anxiety.

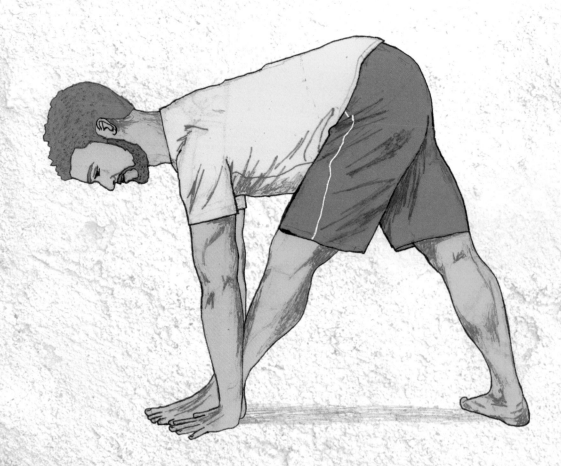

HOW TO DO IT

1 Start in Mountain Pose (see pp. 60–1) with your feet hip-distance apart.

2 Step your right foot towards the back of your mat, turning your toes at a 45-degree angle and the sole of your foot grounded to the mat.

3 Straighten both legs with a micro-bend at your knees.

4 Put your hands on your hips and turn your torso to align with your left foot.

5 Place your fingers or palms to the floor either side of your front foot, or on blocks. Slightly rounding your spine for this is okay.

6 Inhale as you lengthen your spine. Exhale as you hinge forwards from your hips, lowering your chest towards your left thigh.

7 Stay here for five deep, slow breaths. On each inhale, lengthen your spine, creating a flat back. On every exhale, fold a little deeper.

8 Inhale to come up. Repeat on the opposite side.

○ WATCH YOUR FORM

Make sure your feet are hip-distance apart, as it's easier to balance this way.

Ensure you have square hips. This means keeping your torso aligned with your front leg, so you're stretching your hamstrings effectively.

Not hinging properly at the hips is another common issue in this pose. Keep your spine lengthened, paying special attention to your lower back, ensuring it remains in a neutral position.

○ HOW TO MODIFY IT

If you're struggling to balance, taking a wider than hip-distance stance will give you more stability.

A variation for this pose is to interlock your fingers behind your back.

↑ NEXT LEVEL

For a deep shoulder stretch, try this: As you fold forwards from the hips, interlock your hands and draw your them up and over your head. Don't forget to breathe!

Warrior Point

Inversion postures help the flow of oxygenated blood to your sensory organs, which is said to help cognitive function. So if you want to clear your head, bend forward!

WIDE-LEGGED FORWARD FOLD

PRASARITA PADOTTANASANA

(prah-suh-REE-tuh pah-doh-tahn-AHS-uh-nuh)

Whether you're a desk jockey, cyclist or a runner, your body will appreciate the deep stretch that comes with this posture. Wide-Legged Forward Fold is an accessible forward bend for beginners that stretches your hamstrings, lower back, hips and calves.

This posture is also a mild inversion, meaning your head will hang lower than your heart, which is good for calming your mind.

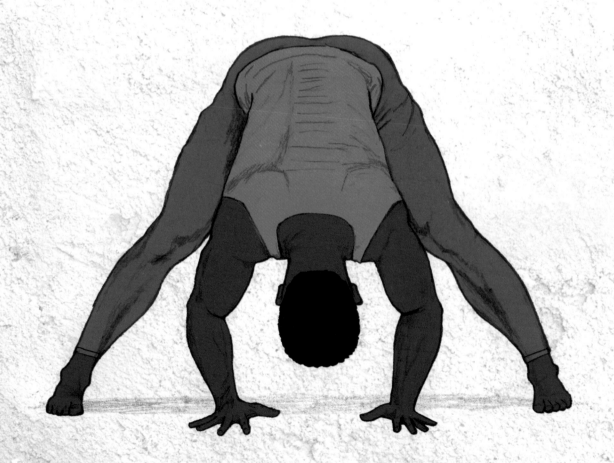

HOW TO DO IT

1 Start in Mountain Pose (see pp. 60–1). Bring your hands on to your hips. Step your feet wide apart with your toes pointing straight ahead.

2 Ensure both the balls and heels of your feet are firmly grounded to the floor.

3 Inhale as you lift your chest and lengthen your spine.

4 Exhale as you hinge forwards from your hips, maintaining a lengthened spine. The aim here is to keep the front of your torso long.

5 Bring your hands to the floor.

6 Relax your head, gazing between your legs.

7 Activate your quads, drawing them upwards. Shift your weight slightly into your heels.

8 Stay here for five slow, deep breaths. With each inhale, lengthen your spine. With each exhale, fold deeper, bringing the top of your head further towards the floor.

9 Inhale and slowly lift your torso upright, maintaining a lengthened spine as you do.

⭘ WATCH YOUR FORM

One common issue in this pose is not maintaining a lengthened torso. Think about creating length in the front of your torso rather than just dropping your head towards the floor.

Make sure you are folding from the hips instead of from the waist. Bring your hands on to your hip bones and hinge from there.

Hyperextending your knees is not advised. It's much better to maintain a micro-bend in your knee joint as this engages all of the muscles around the joint for support.

⭘ HOW TO MODIFY IT

If you have extremely tight hamstrings, you will need two yoga bricks to place your hands on. You could also bend your knees more to reach the floor.

If you're very flexible in your hamstrings, try a more narrow stance.

↑ NEXT LEVEL

The end goal here is to rest the top of your head on the floor while still maintaining a lengthened spine.

Warrior Point

Inversions are effective for spinal realignment, reducing nerve pressure and easing stress.

John's story

John had two small children and a very demanding career as a secondary school teacher when he discovered the power of yoga. He was 38, a keen amateur sportsman whose consumption of beer had risen in inverse proportion to his time spent playing football. He wasn't feeling great and, after yet another gruelling work-week, he decided to accompany his wife to a beginner's yoga class.

Before he knew it John was hooked, and started attending twice-weekly classes. He loved how yoga cleared his mind and stretched his body. For a while, it was the answer to all his stress. But with his time-poor lifestyle, yoga classes eventually became an added demand: getting to class, doing the class, and rushing home afterwards all became too much.

Aged 42, John's life hit crisis point. Not only was his body ragged from the demands of working long hours and fatherhood, but he was now in the middle of a divorce. After admitting that he was burnt out, John took a year off work to recalibrate and recuperate. It was during this year that he met Caleb, and encountered Sattva yoga, a fusion of asana (postures), pranayama (breath-work), kriya (moving chants) and meditation.

At first John was cynical about the 'woo woo' nature of spiritually focused yoga, and felt unsure about the chanting and breath-work. But gradually it became these things that he found most compelling – the way they combined with the strong asana practice offered him a fresh and immersive yoga experience.

John came through his burnout with a better perspective and a solid yoga practice. He realised that the wonderful effects of the yoga he had known actually supported his time and energy, rather than draining it. Sattva yoga was immersive and holistic. For John, it was better than meditation. He loved that it gave him verve and a sense of stillness; how it enabled him to focus completely on the moment without any interference from stressful thoughts.

From time to time John still gets overwhelmed by work, and some weeks the only exercise he gets is when he's walking his dog. He always finds a way to roll out the yoga mat eventually though – because he quietly knows the practice will set him back on his way.

INVERSIONS

As we have discussed, an inversion is a pose in which your heart is higher from the ground than your head. In other words, you're upside down! Aside from literally gaining a fresh perspective there are many health benefits that come with regular inversion practice. They lengthen and strengthen your musculoskeletal system, while stimulating circulation and the lymphatic system. Most importantly, turning yourself upside down oxygenates your brain, which increases memory and focus.

DOWNWARD-FACING DOG

ADHO MUKHA SVANASANA

(Ah-doh MOO-kuh shvan-AHS-uh-nuh)

Easily one of the best-known yoga postures is Downward-Facing Dog. This is the ultimate full-body stretch, lengthening your hamstrings, calves and spine while strengthening and opening your shoulders as you hold yourself in a partial inversion.

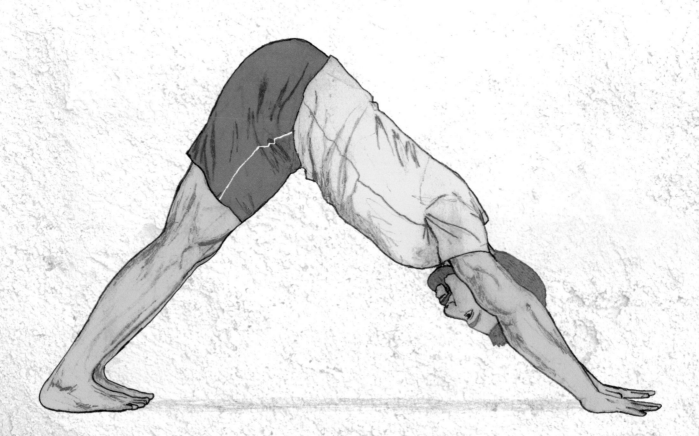

1 Bring yourself on to your hands and knees into tabletop position (see p. 43). Place your knees directly under your hips and your hands directly under your shoulders. Spread your fingers wide and press them into the mat, ensuring that your weight is evenly distributed across your entire hands. This forms a solid foundation for the posture.

2 Now externally rotate your upper arms – biceps facing the front of your mat, triceps facing the back.

3 Tuck your toes under. Exhale as you lift your knees off the mat, sending your hips up and back.

4 Push the floor away from you as you reach your chest towards your thighs.

5 Start to straighten your legs and sink your heels towards the floor. The aim here is to lengthen your spine, so keep your knees bent if you need to.

6 Engage your quads, rotating your thighs inwards as you keep lifting your hips towards the sky.

7 Gaze towards your feet, relaxing your head and neck.

8 Stay here for five deep, slow breaths.

9 Exhale and lower to hands and knees.

○ WATCH YOUR FORM

Make sure your back is not rounded. To lengthen your spine, reach your chest towards your thighs, lifting your butt towards the sky.

Incorrect foot positioning is another common issue here. Your feet should be hip-width apart with your toes pointing towards the front of the mat. Be sure to actively press your heels to the floor.

This is not to say you must have your heels on the floor, since tightness in your hamstrings or calves can make this challenging. It's okay to have your knees bent, so long as you still press your heels towards the floor.

○ HOW TO MODIFY IT

If your hamstrings are tight, keeping your knees bent while lifting your hips high will make it easier to maintain a lengthened spine. As your flexibility improves you will be able to straighten your legs and plant your heels on the mat.

↑ NEXT LEVEL

Try a One-Legged Down Dog, by sweeping your right leg to the sky as high as you can. Maintain a full extension of your leg while keeping your shoulders square. Repeat on the opposite side. Don't forget to breathe!

Warrior Point

You are sort of upside down for this posture, which stimulates the lymphatic and cardiovascular systems and literally gives you a fresh, new perspective.

HALF SHOULDER STAND
ARDHA SARVANGASANA
(ARD-uh shar-vahn-GAHS-uh-nuh)

Spend a lot of time walking or standing? This posture helps to soothe tired legs and achy feet while gently stretching your upper back and neck muscles. It's often practised towards the end of a class as it aids relaxation and lowers blood pressure. Balancing your legs over your head encourages blood flow and lymphatic drainage – all crucial in maintaining a healthy, functioning immune system.

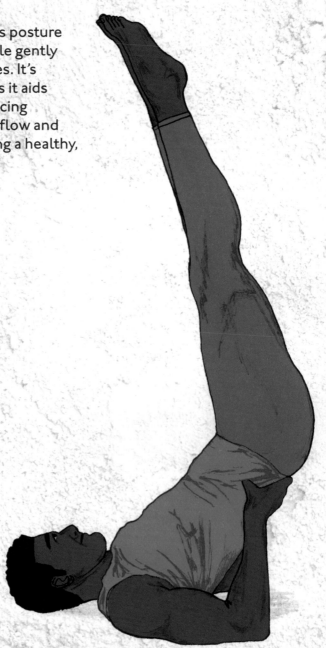

HOW TO DO IT

1 Start by lying down on your back with your knees bent and your arms along the sides of your body, palms pressing into the floor.

2 Inhale deeply. Then, as you exhale, roll your hips up and back towards your chest, bringing your knees above your face.

3 Support your lower back with your hands, elbows on the mat, shoulder-width apart.

4 Extend your legs upwards, drawing them together with flexed feet, toes pointed towards the ceiling.

5 Walk your hands further up your back for extra support. This will bring your chest closer to your chin and open up your back more.

6 Find the place where you can balance your legs over your head with little effort.

7 Stay here for five deep, slow breaths.

8 Exhale as you bend your knees down to your head and slowly, with control, roll your spine to the floor.

○ WATCH YOUR FORM
Avoid placing pressure on your neck and head – instead, you should feel it against your shoulders and upper arms.

Keep hugging your elbows in towards each other to stop them splaying out to the sides.

○ HOW TO MODIFY IT
If you have kyphosis (extreme curvature of the upper back) then you should support your neck with a folded towel or small cushion.

If lifting your legs over your head is a challenge, try using a wall for assistance. Start with your feet at the base of the wall then walk them up until your knees are at 90 degrees. Supporting your lower back, extend one leg at a time over your head.

↑ NEXT LEVEL
Bring your legs to a vertical position to extend into a full shoulder stand.

Warrior Point

Inversions are brain food. With your body upside down, blood rushes to your head, increasing oxygen to your brain. This improves cognitive function. Now that's something to think about!

BRIDGE

SETU BANDHA SARVANGASANA

(SAY-too BAHN-duh shar-vahn-GAHS-uh-nuh)

A calming and beginner-friendly backbend that opens and stretches all the muscles along the front of your body, including your chest, shoulders, abdomen, hips and thighs while strengthening those muscles required to support you in the posture – your back, glutes, legs and ankles.

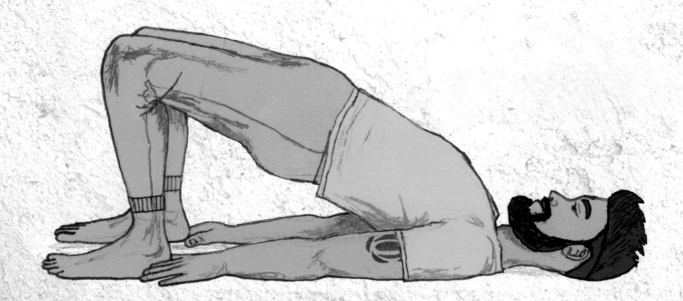

HOW TO DO IT

1 Lie on your back with your knees bent and feet hip-width apart. Extend your arms and wiggle your fingers – your feet should be placed just out of reach of your fingertips.

2 Keep your arms alongside your body, palms pressing into the floor.

3 Maintain your neck in a neutral position so that you're gazing up towards the sky.

4 Draw your shoulder blades back and down.

5 Press your feet into the floor. Inhale as you lift your hips towards the sky, engaging your glutes and hamstrings.

6 Keep your core muscles switched on but your head and neck relaxed.

7 Think about keeping the inner thigh muscles working, so your knees don't drop out sideways.

8 One option is to clasp your hands together below your pelvis, interlocking your fingers. Keep your arms extended and externally rotated. If this is challenging for you, it's okay to keep your palms pressed into the floor shoulder-width apart.

9 Stay here for five deep breaths.

10 Exhale as you slowly roll your spine back to the floor.

WATCH YOUR FORM

When pressing your hips to the sky, be sure to fully engage your hamstrings and glutes – otherwise you will use your lower back muscles instead, which adds unwanted strain.

Be careful not to push your hips too high – this means you're hyperextending your lumbar spine.

Keep your feet, knees and hips in line with one another. Try squeezing a yoga brick between your knees to prevent them dropping outwards.

HOW TO MODIFY IT

If you need lower back support, position a yoga block under your tailbone. You can stand the block at three different heights depending on what position feels most comfortable for you.

↑ NEXT LEVEL

To test your glute strength and hip stability, try extending one leg towards the sky as you maintain your hips at an even level. Ground your standing foot into the floor to stabilise.

Warrior Point

Bridge posture broadens the chest and lifts you up so, in yogi terms, it's a heart-opener. True warriors keep their hearts open, even when things get tough.

Samayan's story

Samayan was 19 years old when he took part in his first gaming competition. He had practised the new strategy game in question for six months and now, here he was – a wild card – challenging pros and raising eyebrows. Before long, he had qualified for World Finals, and found himself flown from England to compete in South Korea. Next thing he knew, Samayan was a professional. Now he had personal contracts – and a salary.

In the world of gaming, he became famous. And for a while, it was amazing. Winning felt incredible, particularly as the underdog. Once his reputation grew, however, he was expected to win, and the pressure on his shoulders was intense. To stay at the top of his game, Samayan had to practise 12 hours per day. It was lonely, stressful – and tough on his body.

When his first love came to a tumultuous ending, Samayan found himself heartbroken and his game started to decline. Soon he was virtually unemployed. Now what?, he thought.

Deciding on a career change, he qualified as a Personal Trainer and dedicated himself to the world of fitness. And then along came a pandemic. The gyms closed and Samayan was stuck. He decided to use the opportunity for spiritual growth and booked himself into an online yoga class. Friends and colleagues had mentioned yoga, but he had always preferred a hard gym workout. Now locked down in his living room, he had nothing left to lose.

It was with optimism that Samayan assumed his first Down Dog, feeling the power of the practice immediately. Not just in his body (his opened shoulders and loosened back) but in mind and spirit too. A few more classes, and he felt amazing. But then one day he just dropped his yoga routine and within weeks he'd fallen back into becoming the man he didn't want to be any more.

If Samayan had needed proof of the power of yoga, then surely this was it. He was astonished at how fast he'd returned to his old patterns of behaviour, and therefore committed himself to an hour's yoga every morning after waking. Yet again, Samayan felt better. Yet again, he could sense the growth. No doubt about it now: when he practised yoga, Samayan felt more connected. Both to himself and something more.

Yoga became not just a physical practice but more a journey into himself, allowing him to access those more sensitive parts of himself that he was taught to hide away. For Samayan, now 27, yoga is a way of 'raising his vibration', helping him tap into universal consciousness. With that, he's discovered a new sense of balance. This balance (seeking it, finding it, cherishing it) is where true manhood lies. Just one year after trying his first ever class, Samayan set his mind on becoming a yoga teacher so he can pass on all he's learned to other men who aren't sure about getting on the mat. Yoga is not just for himself.

FLOOR

Floor Poses can be either strong and challenging or soft and gentle. They include arm balances, which are great for increasing shoulder stability, core strength and stamina; Prone Poses (lying on your belly), which build strength in your lower back and abs, and Supine Poses (lying on your back), which involve twisting, lengthening and relaxing.

PLANK

KUMBHAKASANA

(koom-bahk-AHS-uh-nuh)

This one is the daddy of all core-strengthening postures! Plank targets the deepest abdominal muscles. It works the shoulders, chest, arms, wrists and fingers too. Holding yourself in this high push-up position builds stamina and endurance while also increasing heat and energy throughout your entire body. Plank is also the gateway to building strength for the more challenging arm-balancing postures.

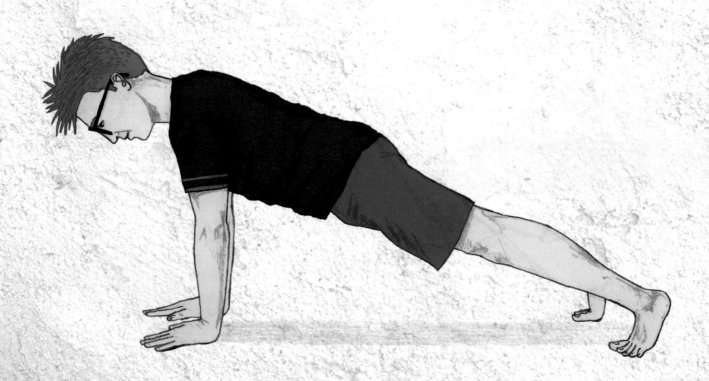

HOW TO DO IT

1 Begin on all fours in a tabletop position (see p. 43). Make sure your shoulders are stacked over your wrists and your arms straightened. Spread your fingers wide and press them into the floor.

2 Step your feet to the back of the mat, keeping them hip distance apart and tucking under your toes. Next, bring your body into a straight line, from your crown to your heels.

3 Draw your navel in towards your spine and tuck in your pelvis.

4 Gently gaze at the floor between your hands while keeping your neck in a neutral position.

5 Externally rotate your upper arms so that your triceps face the back of the mat and your biceps face the front.

6 Push the floor away from you and notice your shoulder blades spreading away from your spine.

7 Engage the muscles on the front of your thighs and press your heels towards the back of your mat.

8 Stay here for five deep, slow breaths. Exhale as you lower your knees to the floor.

WATCH YOUR FORM

Is your lower back sagging? Check that you are maintaining a strong, neutral spine and keeping your back straight.

Another common mistake is not activating your quadriceps. Make sure these muscles are switched on as they support your lower back.

HOW TO MODIFY IT

If you're struggling to hold your entire body weight up, you can always lower your knees to the floor into Half Plank Pose. Be sure to keep your pelvis tucked in to maintain a neutral spine. Continue pushing the floor away from you to ensure full upper body engagement.

↑ NEXT LEVEL

To increase the challenge to your core muscles, try lifting one leg off the mat and hold for three to five breaths. Repeat on the opposite leg.

Still too easy? (Then you're doing great!) Try extending your opposite arm and leg and hold for as long as you are able.

Warrior Point

Plank is pure warrior. It develops presence, focus and concentration.

97

SIDE PLANK

VASISTHASANA

(VAH-shees-THAH-suh-nuh)

Put your balance to the test with this challenging
posture that requires you to stabilise on one arm,
building strength in your shoulders, core, legs, ankles
and wrists. Side Plank is particularly good for toning
your obliques, those muscles on the side of your torso.

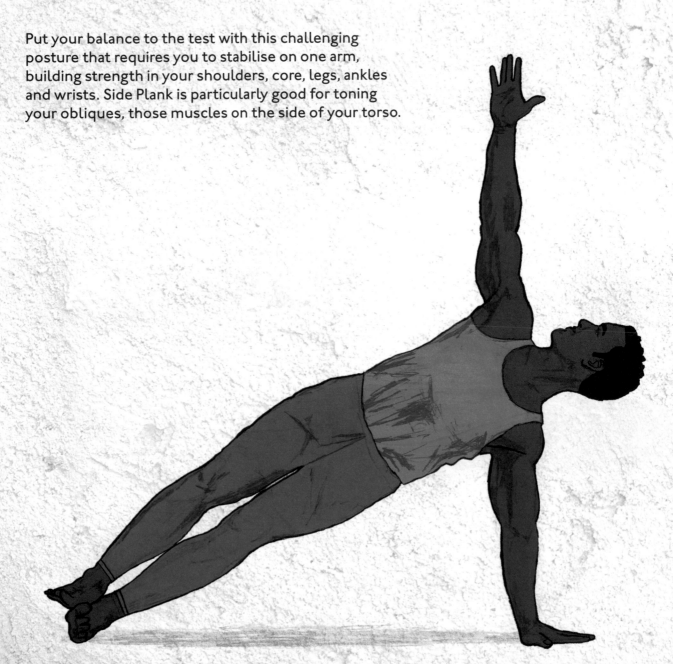

HOW TO DO IT

1 Begin in Plank Pose (see pp. 96–7).

2 Transfer your weight on to your left hand as you roll on to the outer edge of your left foot.

3 Stack your right foot on top of your left.

4 Press into the floor with your left fingers and ensure your left shoulder is stacked over your left wrist.

5 Bring your right hand on to your right hip as you open your chest to stack your shoulders and hips.

6 Focus on lifting your left hip up and maintaining a strong left leg.

7 When you're ready and stable, sweep your right arm up towards the sky, gazing forwards.

8 Stay here for five deep, slow breaths.

9 Exhale and bring your right hand back to the floor, returning to Plank.

10 Repeat on the opposite side.

○ WATCH YOUR FORM

Be sure that your hips are not sagging towards the floor. Keep lifting them up towards the sky, engaging your obliques.

Make sure your pelvis is neither tucked nor arched. Maintain a neutral position.

Don't lock out or hyperextend your elbow on the balancing arm. Keep a micro-bend in the arm to protect the elbow joint and promote stabilisation.

○ HOW TO MODIFY IT

If stacking your feet is too challenging or uncomfortable, you can scissor your legs so that both feet are resting on the floor. Alternatively, you can step your right foot in front of your left shin.

↑ NEXT LEVEL

To take Side Plank up a notch, try extending your top leg towards the sky, keeping your foot flexed and quadriceps fully engaged. Don't forget to breathe!

Warrior Point

Real warriors are supported! This posture adds strength to the obliques and they play a crucial role in keeping your spine strong.

FOUR LIMB STAFF

CHATURANGA DANDASANA

(chah-tuur-ANGH-uh dahn-DAHS-uh-nuh)

A challenging foundational posture that you'll find incorporated into lots of yoga flow sequences, Four Limb Staff is going to test your upper body strength, particularly your shoulders, chest and arms. Mastering this posture will develop your strength for more advanced arm balances.

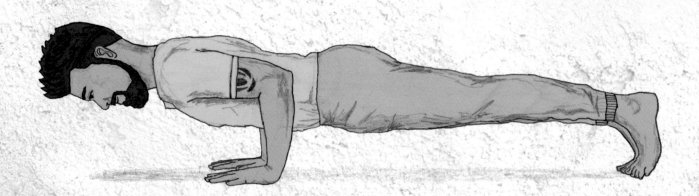

1   Start in Plank position (see pp. 96–7), ensuring your shoulders are stacked over your wrists and your legs extended with quadriceps fully engaged.

2   Your body should be in a straight line, from your crown to your heels, like a plank.

3   Gently gaze at the floor between your hands, while keeping your neck neutral.

4   Externally rotate your upper arms so that your triceps face the back of the mat and your biceps face the front.

5   Shift your weight forwards so that you come on to the tips of your toes. Your shoulders will now be positioned slightly ahead of your wrists.

6   Keep your elbows tucked in to the sides of your ribs. Take a deep breath in, then, as you exhale, slowly lower down, sending your elbows back. Don't allow your elbows to 'wing out' to the sides.

7   Maintain full engagement of your core as you continue to lower until your shoulders are the same height as your elbows. Your upper arms will end up parallel to the floor, with your forearms perpendicular to the floor.

8   Inhale and push back up to Plank.

○ WATCH YOUR FORM

Ensure your shoulders don't drop lower than your elbows as this places strain on your shoulders and wrists. Your body should be in one line from your crown to your heels.

Also, don't let your elbows wing outwards as this is not a traditional push-up.

Maintain a tucked pelvis. Don't allow your butt to stick up in the air!

Don't lower too quickly. A slow, controlled movement is both safer and more challenging.

○ HOW TO MODIFY IT

If you're working on building the upper body strength required for Chaturanga Dandasana, try practising with your knees on the mat. Exhale as you shift your weight forwards, lowering towards the floor until your shoulders move past your wrists. Inhale as you push back to the start position. Repeat three to five times. It won't be long before you're ready to progress to a full Chaturanga.

↑ NEXT LEVEL

Try holding yourself in the low plank position for a few breaths.

Warrior Point

Chaturanga is a powerful pose of surrender, a bowing to nature, life, the sun – all that gives us light, strength and energy, both inside and out.

LOW COBRA

ARDHA BHUJANGASANA

(ARD-uh boo-jahn-GAHS-uh-nuh)

This is your introduction to the world of backbends! Backbending strengthens the muscles that support your spine, which means less back pain, more spinal mobility and a more confident, upright posture.

Low Cobra Pose also strengthens your arms and the front of your shoulders, while stretching your abs, hips and chest.

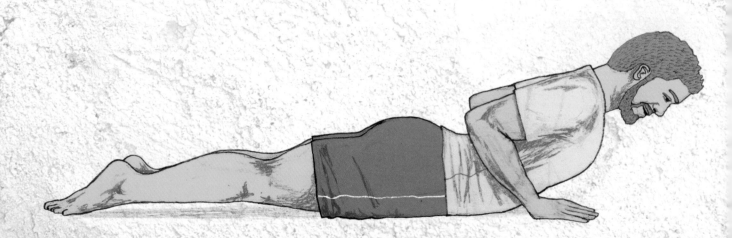

HOW TO DO IT

1 Start by lying face down on your stomach (prone).

2 Place your hands under your shoulders, hugging your elbows into the sides of your ribcage.

3 Gaze down at the mat to ensure your head is in a neutral position.

4 Press your pelvis into the mat.

5 Inhale as you lift your chest off the floor, keeping your lower ribcage connected to the mat.

6 Roll your shoulder blades towards your spine, keeping the elbows hugged towards your ribs (not winging out to the side).

7 Press into the floor with the tops of your feet. Next, squeeze your buttock muscles (glutes). This is really important as it helps support your lower back.

8 Keep your gaze relaxed and focused on the floor.

9 Stay here for five deep, slow, connected breaths.

10 Exhale and slowly release your chest to the floor.

○ WATCH YOUR FORM

Be careful not to hyperextend or strain your neck in any way. The best way to do this is to keep your chin tucked towards your chest – this ensures a neutral spine.

Don't make the mistake of putting too much pressure into your hands. Instead, use your lower back muscles to lift your chest away from the floor.

Make sure you keep your pelvis and legs grounded to the mat. This creates an anchor to allow your chest to lift up.

○ HOW TO MODIFY IT

Feeling pressure in your lower back? Try positioning your feet wider apart, bringing each foot to the edge of the mat. This will alleviate any lower back compression.

To increase your range of movement, try 'rolling your cobra' by lifting your chest on the inhale, lowering on the exhale, and repeating three or four times, like tiny push-ups. With each repetition, see if you can lift the chest a little higher.

↑ NEXT LEVEL

Try lifting your chest off the floor while hovering your hands above the mat. This requires deep glute and lower back muscle activation. Don't forget to breathe!

Warrior Point

Snakes (including cobras) are often perceived as dangerous and deadly but symbolically they represent rebirth, transformation and healing.

COBRA

BHUJANGASANA

(boo-jahn-GAHS-uh-nuh)

Cobra Pose is an energising backbend that stretches the front of your body, opening your chest, shoulders and hips. It also uses muscles in the arms, back and legs in order to arc your spine upwards.

Only progress to this intermediate pose once you've mastered Low Cobra (see page xx) as it's a much deeper extension of the lumbar spine.

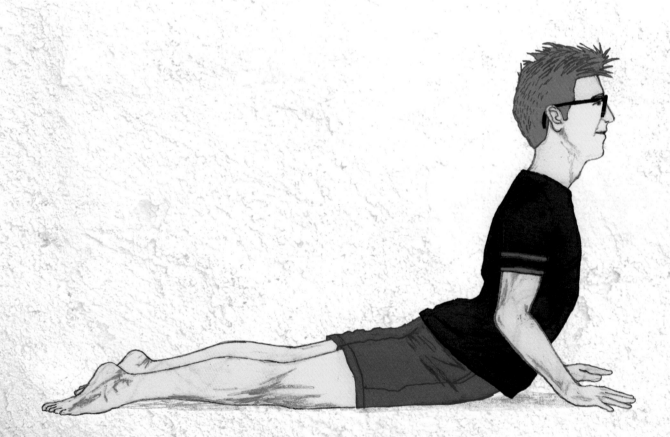

HOW TO DO IT

1 Start by lying face down on your stomach (prone).

2 Place your hands under your shoulders, hugging your elbows into the sides of your ribcage.

3 Gaze down at the mat to ensure your head is in a neutral position.

4 Press your pelvis into the mat.

5 Inhale as you start to straighten your arms, lifting your chest off the floor, as though you're pushing the floor away from you.

6 Roll your shoulder blades towards and down your spine while lifting your chest up.

7 Your elbows should be slightly bent and pointing backwards.

8 Press into the floor with the tops of your feet as you engage your hamstrings and glutes.

9 Lift your chin slightly and maintain a gentle gaze.

10 Stay here for five deep, slow breaths.

11 Exhale and slowly release your chest to the floor.

○ WATCH YOUR FORM

The positioning of your hands is important: make sure they're directly beneath your shoulders (if you place them too far forwards you will end up with your shoulders up around your ears).

Be careful not to lock out your elbows – this can place strain on your elbow and wrist joints. Instead maintain a slight bend of your elbows, keeping them pointing behind you, not winging out to the side.

Be aware of your neck and jaw, to make sure you aren't straining either.

○ HOW TO MODIFY IT

Feeling pressure in your lower back? Try positioning your feet wider apart, bringing each foot to the edge of the mat. This will alleviate any lower back compression.

If you find Cobra a bit hard right now, try Low Cobra.

↑ NEXT LEVEL

Upward-Facing Dog (see pp. 106–7) is the next step up from Cobra, where your thighs and hips are lifted off the floor and your elbows straighten, extending your spine into a deeper backbend.

Warrior Point

Think of a cobra when it rears up. Pretty fearless, right? This posture builds strength in the spine, opens up the chest and elevates the heart.

UPWARD-FACING DOG

URDHVA MUKHA SVANASANA

(OORD-vuh MOO-kuh shvan-AHS-uh-nuh)

This iconic posture is one step up from Cobra – an invigorating backbend practised repeatedly in any yoga flow class. It will strengthen and mobilise your spine, while stretching your chest, shoulders, abdominals and hip flexors.

The main difference between Cobra and Upward-Facing Dog is that the latter strengthens your arms and wrists as you lift and hold your thighs and hips off the floor.

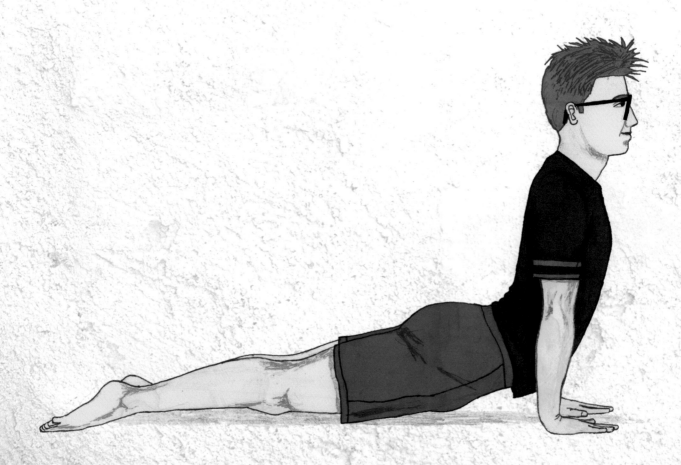

HOW TO DO IT

1   Start in prone position (lying on your stomach).

2   Place your hands close to your ribcage, stacked beneath your elbows. Keep the elbows tucked in, tight, to your sides.

3   Inhale as you straighten your arms, lifting your chest forwards and up towards the sky.

4   Press the tops of your feet into the floor as you lift your hips and thighs to hover over the mat. Your hands and the tops of your feet should be the only body parts connected to the floor.

5   Imagine you're pushing the floor away from you as you roll your shoulder blades towards and down your spine. Try to create space between your shoulders and your ears.

6   Ensure your legs and glutes remain active. This supports your lower back.

7   Lift your chin slightly and maintain a gentle gaze.

8   Stay here for five deep, slow breaths.

9   Exhale as you lower down to the floor, returning to a prone position.

WATCH YOUR FORM

If your shoulders are up around your ears, then you're doing this incorrectly. Keep your back engaged and aim to move your shoulder blades down your spine.

Are you craning your neck? This is called hyperextension, which can cause aches and strains. To maintain the natural curvature of your neck, gaze gently ahead.

Are your knees touching the mat? The goal here is to fully activate your thighs to lift your legs off the floor. And, as Upward-Facing Dog is such a deep backbend, engagement of your glutes is essential for lower back support.

HOW TO MODIFY IT

If lifting your hips and thighs off the floor feels too hard, then switch your Upward-Facing Dog for Cobra.

Warrior Point

Be like a loyal dog to your practice. Show up every day. With persistence and dedication, you will be rewarded.

LOCUST

SALABHASANA

(shah-lah-BAHS-uh-nuh)

Locust is a beginner's backbend and an energy-booster. It strengthens all of the muscles along the posterior of your body, including back, glutes, triceps, core, thighs and calves.

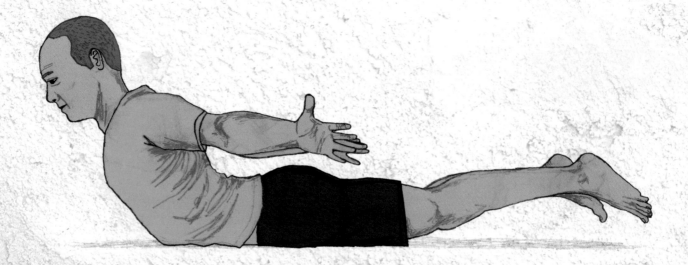

HOW TO DO IT

1 Lie on your belly with your arms along your sides, palms facing down. Keep your forehead resting gently on the mat.

2 Draw your navel in towards your spine. Roll your shoulders back, drawing your shoulder blades together.

3 Inhale and lift your head, chest and arms off the floor, while also lifting your legs up too.

4 Fully lengthen your arms, pointing your fingers towards your toes. Keep moving your shoulder blades down your spine.

5 Engage your glutes but do not let your pelvis come off the mat.

6 Extend and engage your legs while pointing your toes.

7 Keep your head in a neutral position, gently gazing at the floor. Relax your face, relax your eyes.

8 And breathe! Five deep, slow breaths.

9 Exhale and release to the floor. Rest your head to one side.

10 When you're ready, repeat. Then repeat again!

○ WATCH YOUR FORM

Overextending your neck can cause unnecessary strain. Keep your neck lengthened and your head in a neutral position.

Bending the knees might feel tempting but don't do it: it just puts pressure on your lower back.

Relaxing your belly also compromises your lower back. Keep drawing your navel towards your spine at all times.

○ HOW TO MODIFY IT

If your lower back hurts or feels uncomfortable, perform this posture with both legs resting on the mat. From there you can try lifting one leg at a time, while keeping both hips grounded to the floor.

Another easier option is to keep your palms connected to the mat while keeping the triceps engaged.

↑ NEXT LEVEL

Instead of pointing your fingers towards your toes, try interlocking them behind your lower back for a deeper chest stretch.

For a bigger core challenge, extend your arms in front of you with fingers reaching forwards and palms down.

Warrior Point

Locust Pose activates your solar plexus, the seat of your passion, optimism and willingness to go beyond.

WIND-RELIEVING POSE

PAVANAMUKTASANA

(pah-van-ah-mook-TAHS-uh-nuh)

This gentle and relaxing pose will release tension in your lower back and abdomen while massaging your internal organs. And yes, this posture gets its name from its efficacy to make you pass wind – best practised alone!

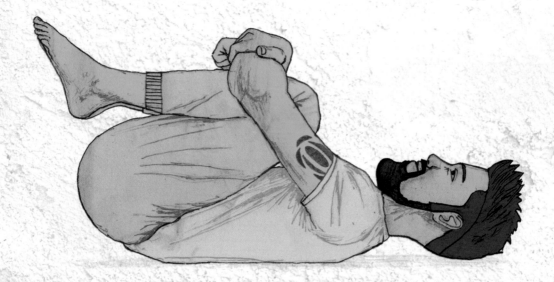

1 Lie on your back with your legs extended and arms by your side.

2 Inhale, then as you exhale bend your knees and bring your thighs to your belly.

3 Wrap your arms around your legs, drawing your knees to your chest.

4 Stay here for five slow, connected breaths.

○ WATCH YOUR FORM

Make sure your neck is relaxed and neutral by keeping your chin tucked in. Use a rolled-up blanket or yoga brick to support your head if you need it.

○ HOW TO MODIFY IT

If you can't reach your knees, wrap a yoga strap or a towel around them and draw your knees towards your chest.

   If your hips are very tight, try practising with one leg at a time. Begin with both knees bent, feet on the floor. Draw your right knee to your chest. Then repeat on the opposite side.

↑ NEXT LEVEL

For a deeper spinal stretch, try bringing your nose towards your knees.

Warrior Point

Gently massaging your intestines is beneficial for your digestive health. And remember, it's only air!

SUPINE LEG STRETCH

SUPTA PADANGUSTHASANA

(SOOP-tah pahd-ahng-goosh-TAHS-uh-nuh)

This is a classic stretch for relieving tension in all of the muscles that run up the back of your legs and into your lower back. Tight hamstrings often lead to tight calves, which can lead to tight Achilles tendons. This tightness can affect your walking and running gait, which can lead to injuries, particularly while playing any kind of sport.

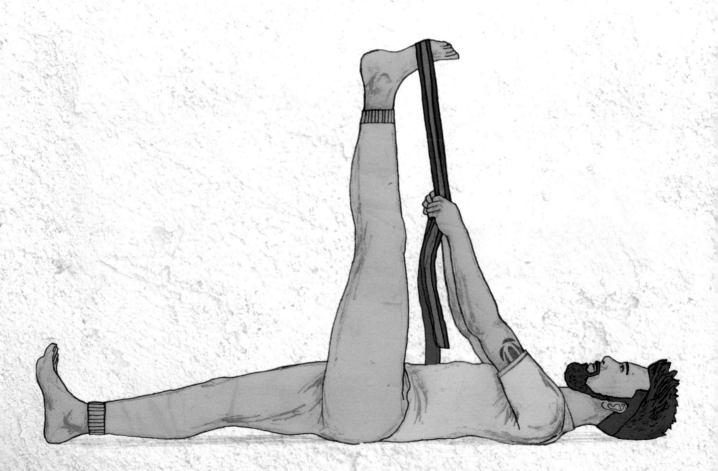

1 Start by lying on your back with your legs extended.

2 Bend your left leg towards your chest and hook your yoga strap (or belt) around the ball of your foot. Hold the strap in each hand as you flex your foot.

3 Extend your leg to where it feels slightly uncomfortable. If you can't straighten your leg to a perpendicular position, that's okay.

4 Keep flexing your foot, pointing your toes towards your knee and pressing your heel towards the sky. Keep both glutes grounded to the mat, while relaxing your neck and shoulders.

5 Stay here for five deep, controlled breaths. With every exhalation, deepen a little further into the stretch.

6 Exhale and slowly release your left leg to the floor. Repeat on the opposite side.

○ WATCH YOUR FORM

Ensure your upper back and the back of your head remain connected to the mat to avoid neck strain.

Don't allow the hip of the lifting leg to ride up off the floor. Instead, keep both glutes equally pressed into the mat.

○ HOW TO MODIFY IT

If you have lower back issues, rather than extending the resting leg on the mat, try bending your knee with your foot flat. This reduces the load on your lumbar spine.

If your neck is hyperextended while lying on the floor, you can support your head with a yoga brick or a cushion.

↑ NEXT LEVEL

If you can maintain your leg extended at a 90-degree angle, then try pulling your foot further towards your head.

To stretch the muscles of your inner and outer thighs, as well as your hamstrings, take the strap in your right hand and slowly lower your right leg out to the right side. Return to centre, then take the strap with your left hand and slowly lower your leg out to the left. Repeat on the other side.

Warrior Point

As any sportsman will attest, supple hamstrings give you the power to do your best.

SUPINE TWIST
SUPTA MATSYENDRASANA
(SOOP-tah MAHT-see-en-DRAHS-uh-nuh)

Here's a soothing spinal rotation that's often done at the end of a session to relax your body, calm the nervous system and cultivate a grounded energy.

Supine Twist gently stretches the muscles in your mid to lower back, your shoulders, chest, obliques and glutes.

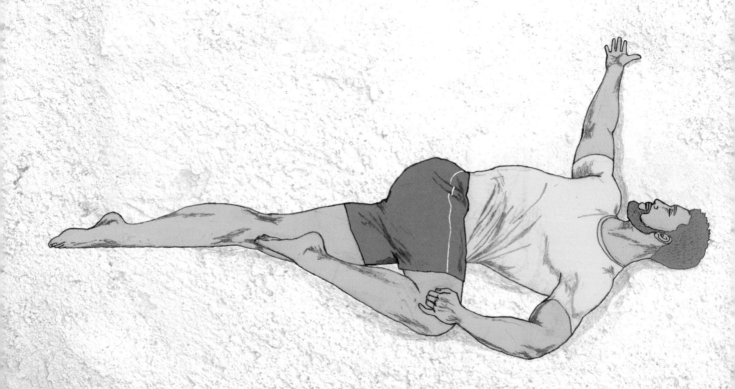

HOW TO DO IT

1 Lie on your back with your legs bent and feet on the floor.

2 Draw both knees towards your chest.

3 Extend your left leg and rest it on the mat, keeping your right knee to your chest and holding it with your left hand.

4 Outstretch your right arm away from your body, gazing towards your right hand.

5 Inhale, then exhale as you gently pull your right knee across the midline of your body towards the floor on the left side.

6 Stay here for five deep, slow breaths. With every exhalation, release your right shoulder and right knee further to the mat.

7 Inhale, returning to centre. Repeat on the opposite side.

○ WATCH YOUR FORM

It's important to keep your shoulder connected to the mat, more so than it is to bring your knee all the way to the floor (if your knee floats up a bit, that's okay).

○ HOW TO MODIFY IT

If your neck is hyperextended while lying on the floor, you can support your head with a yoga brick or a cushion.

If you're really tight in your upper back and neck, you may find neck rotations really challenging. In that case, maintain your head in a neutral position.

For an easier stretch, twist with both knees bent.

↑ NEXT LEVEL

For a deeper stretch, start with both knees bent, feet on the floor. Cross your right knee over your left knee, then gently pull both knees towards the floor on the left side.

Warrior Point

Wring out the tension and stress from your day as you quietly connect body to breath.

PIGEON

EKA PADA RAJAKAPOTASANA

(EKK-uh PAHD-uh RAH-juh-KA-poh-TAHS-uh-nuh)

Lower back issues are one of the biggest health complaints in men. Did you know that tight hips are often the cause? Your hips and pelvis are the foundation to spinal health. Pigeon Pose is the ultimate hip opener. This posture also alleviates tightness in your hamstrings, pelvis, groin and glutes.

   Traditionally, Pigeon Pose is practised towards the end of a class as it prepares your hips and lower back for the seated postures.

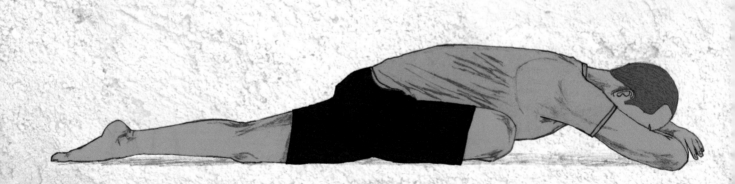

HOW TO DO IT

1 Start in Downward-Facing Dog (see pp. 88–9). Bring your right knee forwards and place it on the outside of your right wrist.

2 Your shinbone should be lying across the mat at a 45-degree angle.

3 Lower your left knee to the mat and untuck your left toes. Make sure your left foot is pointing towards the back of the mat.

4 Square your hips to the front of your mat.

5 You may want to prop a yoga brick or cushion under your right hip for support.

6 Inhale and lengthen your spine. Exhale and fold your torso forwards, resting your forehead on the mat, your hands or a yoga brick.

7 Stay here for five deep, slow breaths.

8 Inhale to come back up on to your hands. Tuck your right toes. Lift your right knee off the mat. Exhale back to Downward-Facing Dog. Repeat on the opposite side.

○ WATCH YOUR FORM

It's important to place your knee at the edge of your mat, outside of your wrist, with your shinbone at a 45-degree angle across the mat.

Make sure you aren't collapsing into the floor with the hip of your bent knee. Use a yoga brick or cushion under your butt on that side for support and keep your hips square with the weight evenly distributed across both hips.

Don't let your back leg rotate outwards. Instead, consciously ensure that your hips are square and that your back leg is in a straight line.

○ HOW TO MODIFY IT

If the forward fold is not accessible for you, you can maintain an upright torso, gently leaning forwards.

You could progress by using blocks to rest your forearms on. Over time you'll eventually reach your forehead to the mat.

↑ NEXT LEVEL

Once you're comfortable in Pigeon Pose, try adding a quad stretch. With your torso upright, bend your left knee and grab your ankle with your left hand. Gently pull your heel towards your butt.

Warrior Point

Supple hips stave off back pain and other injuries as well as having a crossover to other sports and making you a better lover.

CORPSE

SAVASANA

(shah-VAHS-uh-nuh)

This resting pose is where every yoga class ends and is considered to be one of the most challenging postures of all. This is because it requires you to stay still in body and mind. This isn't falling asleep at the end of the class! Savasana requires focus and presence as you allow yourself to relax while remaining alert.

    It may be tempting to skip Savasana but your yoga practice is never complete without it. Think of it as the time required for your body and brain to download everything you've just done.

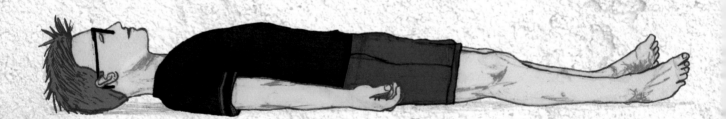

1 Lie down on your back.

2 Separate your legs and allow your feet to drop out to the sides.

3 Position your arms along the sides of your body, slightly away from your torso with your palms facing the sky.

4 Draw your shoulder blades together.

5 Rest your head in a neutral position.

6 Relax all of your limbs, as well as your face. Feel the weight of your body against the floor.

7 Bring your focus to the gentle flow of your breath, in and out through your nose. If your mind starts to wander, bring it back to your breath.

8 Stay here for at least five minutes. Setting an alarm is useful so you don't need to be checking your watch.

9 When you're ready to come out of the pose, reach your arms over your head and take a full body stretch.

10 Bring your knees to your chest and roll over on to your right side. Stay here for a few moments before gently propping yourself upright.

○ WATCH YOUR FORM

Thinking is probably the hardest thing to avoid in this posture! If you struggle to still your mind, bring your focus back to your breath and try this technique: Inhale for four counts, exhale for four counts. This practice will help settle your thoughts, allowing you to relax.

Falling asleep? The aim of Savasana is for the mind to stay awake, but calm. Try to maintain your awareness by observing your breath, body and thoughts without attaching to them.

↑ HOW TO MODIFY IT

If your neck is hyperextended while lying on the floor, you can support it with a yoga brick or a cushion.

If you have lower back issues, place cushions under your slightly bent knees as this will take the pressure off your lumbar curve.

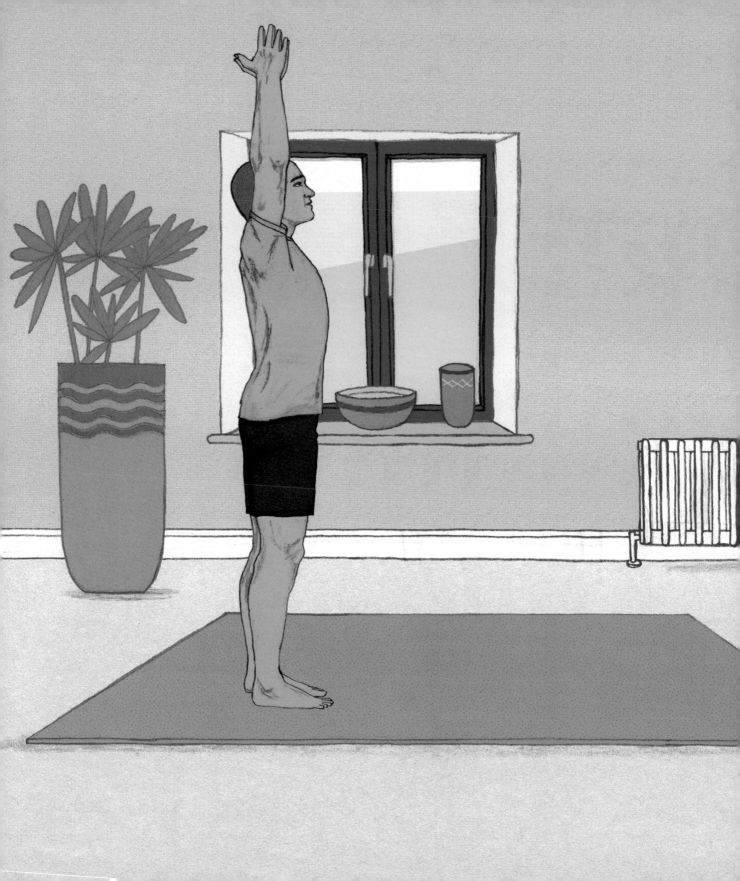

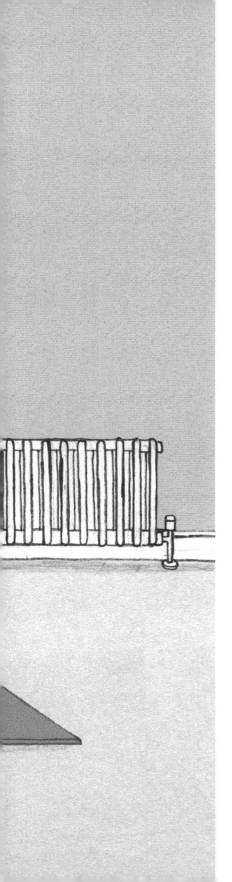

THE VINYASAS

Surya = Sun

Namaskar = to bow or to adore

A Sun Salutation, known as Surya Namaskar, is considered a prayer in motion, a connection between you and the power of the Sun. Traditionally practised as a ritual of gratitude and respect, this sequence of postures, connected to breath, builds heat and strength in your body – igniting the sun within.

Salutations form a solid foundation for your yoga practice. They teach you how to move, breathe and flow between postures, awakening your whole body – physically, mentally and energetically.

Here we'll introduce you to two variations; Surya Namaskar A and Surya Namaskar B. We suggest starting off with a couple of rounds of each, building it up over time as your strength, flexibility and coordination develops.

Experiment with varying the tempo. A faster pace will increase your heart rate, making for a great full-body cardio workout with detoxifying effects. Or try slowing it right down while mindfully giving attention to your body and breath as you move through the various planes of motion.

Whichever way you flow, Sun Salutations are a fantastic way to bring you into a meditative state, unifying mind, body and breath.

SUN SALUTATION A
SURYA NAMASKAR A
(SOOR-yuh nah-muh-SKAR-uh A)

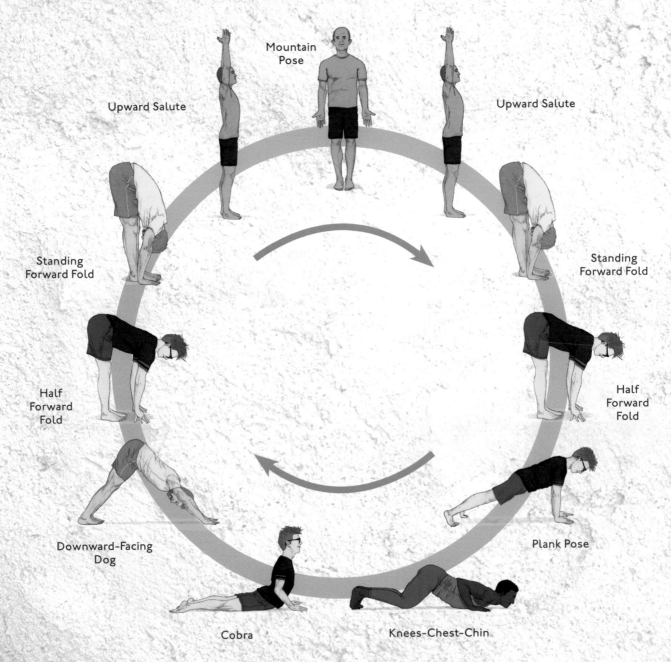

Mountain Pose

Upward Salute

Upward Salute

Standing Forward Fold

Standing Forward Fold

Half Forward Fold

Half Forward Fold

Downward-Facing Dog

Plank Pose

Cobra

Knees-Chest-Chin

HOW TO DO IT

1 Begin in Mountain Pose (see pp. 60–1) with your hands at your heart in prayer position. Inhale as you sweep your arms over your head, arching your back slightly – this is known as Upward Salute. Touch your hands together then exhale to bring your hands into prayer position at your heart as you hinge forwards from your hips.

2 Bring your fingertips to your shins (or the floor if you have the flexibility), as you relax your head, neck and shoulders into Standing Forward Fold.

3 Inhale to lift halfway, lengthening your spine and drawing your navel in to support your lower back – this is known as Half Forward Fold.

4 Exhale as you bend your knees and ground your hands to the floor.

5 Inhale as you step your feet to the back of the mat and come into Plank Pose.

6 Exhale as you lower your knees to the floor, followed by your chest and chin – elbows hugging into your ribs.

7 Untuck your toes, then inhale as you lower your hips to the floor and scoop your chest up to Cobra. Remember to keep your elbows tucked close to your ribs, shoulders blades moving down your spine.

8 On your next exhalation, tuck your toes and send your hips up and backward into Downward-Facing Dog. Push the floor away from you as you reach your chest towards your thighs, lengthening your spine. Stay here for five slow, connected breaths.

9 Inhale as you bend your knees and look forwards. Exhale as you lightly step or jump to the front of your mat to return to Forward Fold. Inhale, bringing your hands to your shins and lift into Half Forward Fold. Exhale and fold.

10 On your next inhalation, ground your feet, soften your knees and sweep your arms up to the sky returning to Upward Salute. As you exhale, return to Mountain Pose with your hands at your heart in prayer position.

SUN SALUTATION B
SURYA NAMASKAR B
(SOOR-yuh nah-muh-SKAR-uh B)

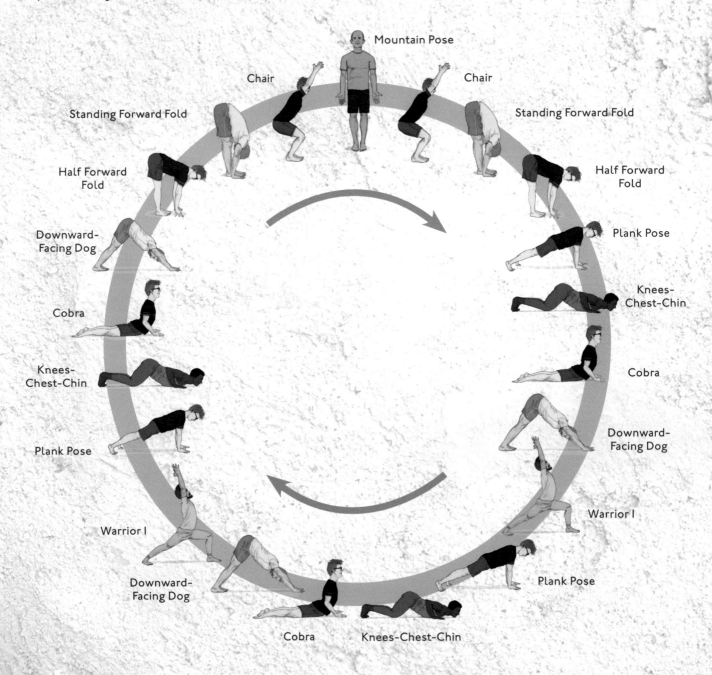

Mountain Pose

Chair

Chair

Standing Forward Fold

Standing Forward Fold

Half Forward Fold

Half Forward Fold

Downward-Facing Dog

Plank Pose

Cobra

Knees-Chest-Chin

Knees-Chest-Chin

Cobra

Plank Pose

Downward-Facing Dog

Warrior I

Warrior I

Downward-Facing Dog

Plank Pose

Cobra

Knees-Chest-Chin

HOW TO DO IT

1 Begin in Mountain Pose (see pp. 60–1) with hands at your heart in prayer position. As you inhale, sweep your arms over your head, bend your knees and come to Chair Pose (see pp. 64–5).

2 Exhale to fold forwards, relaxing your head, neck and shoulders.

3 Inhale to lift halfway, lengthening your spine and drawing your navel in to support your lower back.

4 Exhale as you bend your knees and ground your hands to the floor.

5 Inhale as you step your feet to the back of the mat and come into Plank Pose (see pp. 96–7).

6 Exhale as you lower your knees to the floor, followed by your chest and chin – elbows hugging into your ribs.

7 Untuck your toes, then inhale as you lower your hips to the floor and scoop your chest up to Cobra (see pp. 104–5). Remember, keep your elbows tucked close to your ribs, shoulders blades moving down your spine.

8 On your next exhalation, tuck your toes and send your hips up and back to Downward-Facing Dog (see pp. 88–9).

9 Inhale as you bend your knees and look forwards. Exhale as you step your right foot to the front of the mat, grounding your left heel at 45 degrees.

10 Inhale to sweep your arms overhead, rising up to Warrior I (see pp. 68–9).

11 Exhale as you bring your hands to the floor. Inhale as you step your right foot back to Plank.

12 Exhale as you lower your knees to the floor, followed by your chest and chin. Inhale into Cobra. Exhale to Downward Facing Dog. Then repeat Warrior I on the left side, followed by Plank, Knees-Chest-Chin and Cobra.

13 When you return to Downward Facing Dog, stay here for five slow, connected breaths. Push the floor away from you as you reach your chest towards your thighs, lengthening your spine.

14 Inhale as you bend your knees and look forwards. Exhale as you lightly step or jump to the front of your mat to return to Forward Fold. Inhale, bringing your hands to your shins and lift halfway. Exhale and fold.

15 On your next inhalation, ground your feet, bend your knees and sweep your arms up alongside your ears into Chair Pose. As you exhale, return to Mountain Pose with hands at your heart in prayer position.

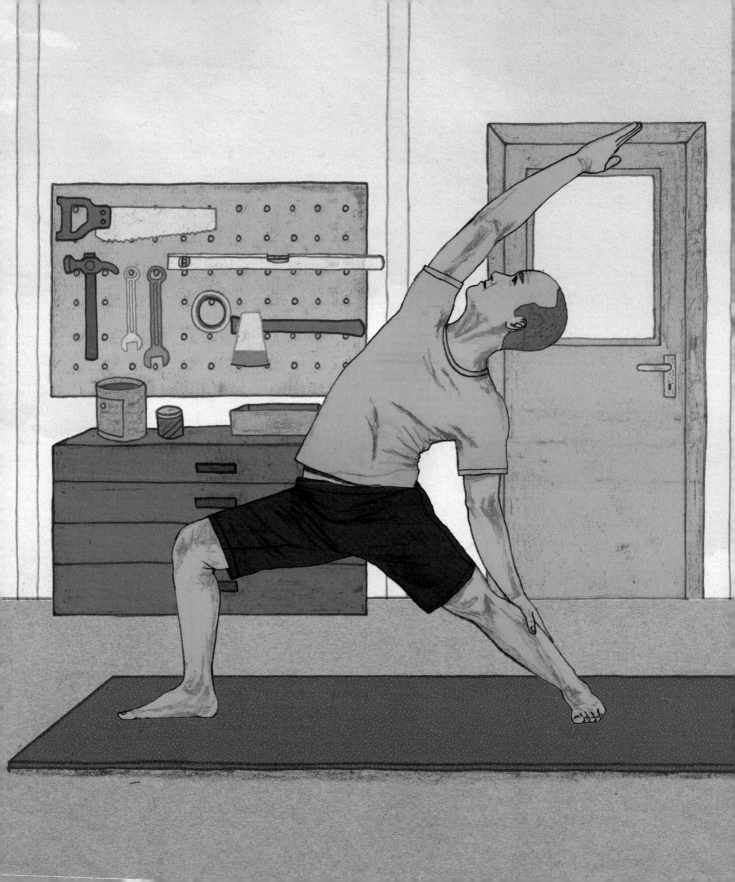

SPIRITUALITY

What does it mean to be spiritual? Must you burn sage and wear cheesecloth clothing? Must you believe in a specific god?

No, is our answer – although you can, if that feels right.

But really, spirituality just involves being connected to human spirit and accessing that part of yourself that exists beyond the physical, beyond what you can experience through your five senses. Spiritual men accept the presence of the biological (yes) but also the inexplicable. They know that we are both a body and a soul, that we are each made up of tangible matter and intangible spirit. Spirituality incorporates and encompasses a huge range of beliefs and teachings, though it's always underpinned by one belief, that we are all consciousness, connected to the Universe, as One.

So how is this all connected to yoga?

Yoga is a spiritual tool, a way for you to tune in to those deeper, intangible aspects of yourself. It helps focus your mind away from the material world and enables you to access deep presence. This is the same level of focus that professional athletes, artists and actors talk about. Here you tap into pure consciousness. You go beyond the body, beyond time, beyond the 'egoic self'. Which makes yoga a doorway to your True Self.

Now let's talk about the ego. In simplistic terms the ego is our mind's construction of who we are. It's something that's often misunderstood as being all bad (or all good) and in fact, it's neither (or both); everybody needs to develop a sufficiently strong ego as they grow in order to feel like a whole person. The problems come when we over-identify with our ego – we think that we are whatever our mind tells us and we end up with a false sense of self. We start to believe that we are our thoughts, our body, our feelings, and not that we are a being and spirit that goes beyond the ego. Most people's egos are fairly fragile too, they seek validation by way of compliments, material goods, popularity and a satisfactory mirror image.

Yoga takes us away from ego and towards spirit. It's about discovering something greater than one's own mind to access and believe in. When your consciousness expands, you're able to transcend the ego (with practice!) and soon begin to realise your unique path and higher purpose.

These are ancient philosophical teachings, and we can promise you, when applied, they work. A regular yoga and meditation practice helps you remember who you really are, which is a man whose mind, heart and spirit are constantly expanding.

MEDITATIONS

TIPS FOR MEDITATING

SETTING

This is about creating the perfect ambience for your meditation. Some call it creating a 'sacred space'. Do you want to light a candle? Burn some incense? What's most important is that there is no clutter, and no distractions. So, before you meditate, be sure to clear away those half-filled coffee mugs and close the door to the background noise.

PREPARATION

Wear loose comfortable clothing. Check the temperature – is it too warm, too cold? Do you need a fan on, or a heater? Switch off your phone and set a timer if you need to. If you live with family or housemates, give them the heads-up you're about to meditate so there will not be interruptions.

POSTURE

It's important to sit tall and upright during meditation as your nervous system runs along your spine. Holding a strong spine allows for energy to flow without obstruction. So that you can comfortably maintain this posture for the duration of your meditation practice, prop yourself up on a bolster or cushion, or simply sit in a chair.

TIMING

Choose the time of day when you're going to be the least distracted. Is it first thing in the morning, before you switch on your phone and check emails? Is it last thing at night, after your day is done? Maybe there's a gap in your schedule when you can slot your meditation in. What matters most is that you are consistent with your meditation practice, and if you miss a day, you get back on it. The magic comes with repeated action, so like brushing your teeth, having a shower and eating your breakfast – just commit to daily meditation.

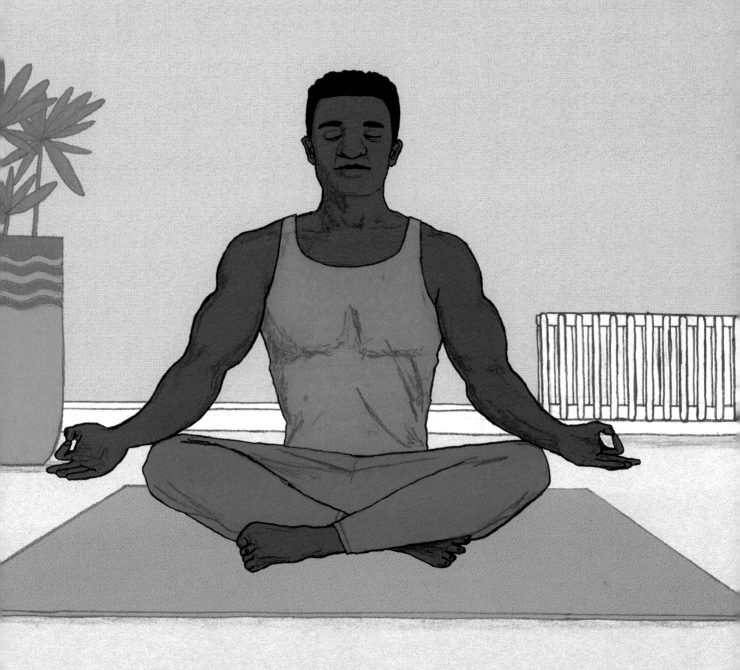

I AM THAT

This meditation will focus your mind on the mystery of being; the notion that you are at one with the universal energy that is constantly supporting you and nourishing you.

As you observe your breath, you will silently chant I AM THAT, THAT I AM, a powerful mantra that means whatever I seek is within me.

This is a great meditation for bringing calm and positivity.

HOW TO DO IT

1 Sit comfortably with an upright, tall spine, either on the floor or in a chair. If you're sitting on the floor, prop yourself up on a cushion to elevate your hips slightly higher than your knees. If you're sitting on a chair, sit forwards so you're not leaning against the back of the chair.

2 Rest your hands on your knees with your palms facing up. Position your chin slightly down to lengthen the back of your neck.

3 Close your eyes and bring your awareness to the tidal rhythm of your breath; the gentle flow of inhalation and exhalation, through your nose.

4 Now, when you are ready, begin to silently chant the mantra. As you inhale, chant I AM THAT. As you exhale, chant THAT I AM.

5 Keep your body and breath relaxed, synchronising the breath and mantra. If your mind starts to wander (perfectly normal, by the way) draw your attention back to the mantra, contemplating its meaning: whatever I seek is within me.

6 Continue for a minimum of five minutes, building up to 15 minutes.

LIGHTNESS OF BEING

For this meditation, you'll use the power of visualisation to develop your awareness of light within your body and bio-magnetic field.

In Sanskrit, Aham Prakasha means 'I Am Light'. As you softly chant this mantra, you'll hold both hands interlocked above your crown while circling your torso.

This alchemy of sound, movement and visualisation will lead you to an internal peaceful state.

HOW TO DO IT

1 Sit comfortably with an upright, tall spine, either on the floor or in a chair. If you're sitting on the floor, prop yourself up on a cushion to elevate your hips slightly higher than your knees. If you're sitting on a chair, sit forwards so you're not leaning against the back of the chair.

2 Bring your hands above your head and interlock your fingers, palms facing down.

3 Close your eyes and begin to circle your torso clockwise while you gently chant AHAM PRAKASHA.

4 As you maintain a seamless, fluid movement, visualise golden light emanating from your crown and circling your body to create a golden sphere.

5 Continue for a minimum of five minutes, building a strong awareness of light emanating from within you and around you.

6 To finish, come to centre and inhale deeply through your nose. As you exhale through your nose, lower your hands to your knees, palms facing up.

THE ART OF TRATAKA

In Sanskrit, Trataka means 'to gaze steadily'. This form of meditation uses the sense of sight to clear clutter from your psyche, developing strong concentration and single pointedness.

Sitting in a darkened room, you'll focus your eyes on a burning candle while trying not to blink. The power of this practice disengages you from mind chatter while strengthening your ability to focus.

HOW TO DO IT

1 Set yourself up in a dimly lit, or darkened room.

2 Position a candle at arm's length away from you, with its flame at eye level, ensuring it doesn't flicker.

3 Sit comfortably with an upright, tall spine, either on the floor or in a chair. If you're sitting on the floor, prop yourself up on a cushion to elevate your hips slightly higher than your knees. If you're sitting on a chair, sit forwards so you're not leaning against the back of the chair.

4 Rest your hands on your knees with your palms facing up. Position your chin slightly down to lengthen the back of your neck.

5 Softly gaze at the candle flame, trying not to blink.

6 Hold this gaze for as long as possible without straining your eyes.

7 When your eyes become watery, close them, holding the image of the flame in your awareness for as long as you can. As the image fades, open your eyes again to continue gazing at the flame.

8 Continue for five to 10 minutes without forcing your concentration. Allow it to happen, naturally, through a relaxed and open mind.

LET IT GO

This is the practice of distinguishing the Self beyond your physicality, age, race, gender, status, beliefs and stories. It is about letting go of repetitive thoughts and labels or judgements, noticing these things as they appear and how they are just mirrors of your mind.

As you practise, you'll become a silent witness to your thoughts, observing them without attaching to them. This technique helps you widen the gap between your thoughts and reactions, facilitating a shift from stress to peace.

HOW TO DO IT

1. Sit comfortably with an upright, tall spine, either on the floor or in a chair. If you're sitting on the floor, prop yourself up on a cushion to elevate your hips slightly higher than your knees. If you're sitting on a chair, sit forwards so you're not leaning against the back of the chair.

2. Rest your hands on your knees with your palms facing up. Position your chin slightly down to lengthen the back of your neck.

3. Close your eyes and bring your awareness to your breath; the gentle flow of inhalation and exhalation, through your nose.

4. As you inhale, feel your navel gliding out, your diaphragm moving down, your lungs expanding. As you exhale, notice the softening of your chest, your diaphragm moving up as your navel moves inwards.

5. Watch your thoughts come and go. See them as gently moving clouds in the sky. They appear, they transform, they disappear.

6. Observe them without any attachment, without attaching emotion to them. See them simply as clouds rather than facts or the truth of things.

7. You may feel sensations in your body. You may hear internal sounds or voices. Acknowledge them without judgement.

8. And let them go.

9. Experience a state of calm as you release anxiousness, tension and chatter from your mind.

10. Continue for five minutes, building up to 20 minutes over time.

WALKABOUT

Often we walk on autopilot, distracted by our internal dialogue and oblivious to our surroundings, and even our bodies. The practice of meditative walking pulls you out of your head and into your physicality, creating stillness of mind.

This is more than just 'a stroll in the park'. It's a multi-sensory experience of creating embodied awareness through movement. If you're a busy or restless guy, this is the ideal meditation for you.

HOW TO DO IT

1 Step outside your front door and pause for a moment. Take a few deep breaths, tuning into your body. Bring your awareness to your feet. Feel the ground beneath you.

2 Start to walk at a slow and even pace – eyes looking ahead. With each step, be aware of the sensations in your feet as they make contact with the ground. Notice how they land. Don't look down, just feel it. Do your heels touch first? Or is it the balls of your feet? Are your feet in the same plane? Or does one of them slightly kick outwards? Where are your knees positioned? What are your hips doing?

3 Just observe, with no judgement. If your mind starts to wander, bring your awareness back into your body, focusing on the physical sensations.

4 Start to pick up your pace a little. Notice your breath. Where are your arms? Are they swinging by your sides? Maybe your hands are in your pockets. Are they warm?

5 Now allow your awareness to expand outwards to your surroundings. Mindfully turn your attention to the natural world. What catches your eye? What colours, shades and textures do you see? Observe and try not to label anything. Just be aware of the aliveness and vibrancy of it all.

6 Tune into that same vibrancy within you. Can you feel it? It's not in your head. It's in your body, pulsating within every cell.

7 Continue the practice for as long as you wish (30 minutes is ideal). To finish, return to a stationary position. Take a few deep, slow breaths, setting an intention to keep this awareness with you while you continue your day.

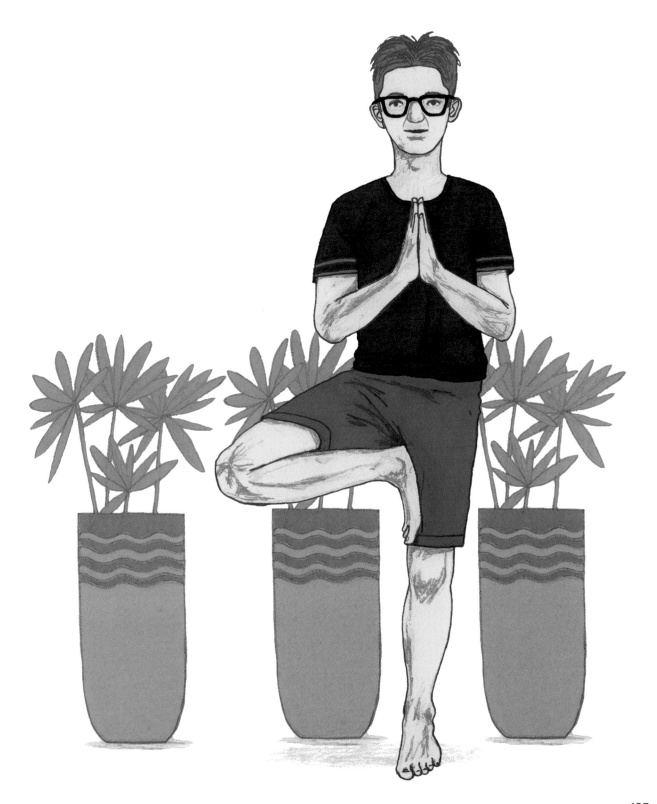

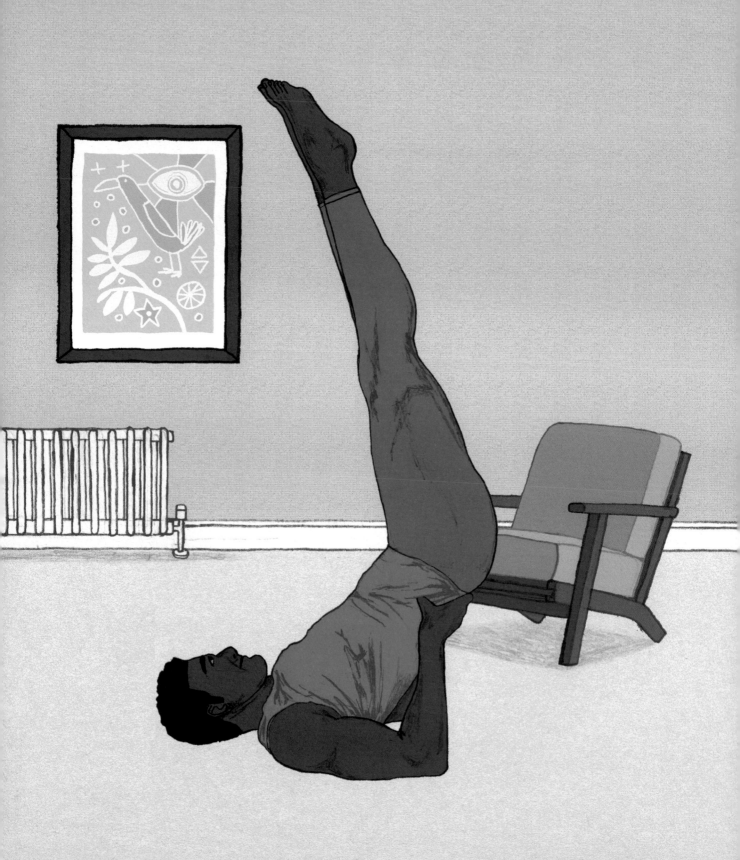

HEART-CENTRED LIVING

Some guys think that walking around with an open heart renders them weak and vulnerable. This could not be further from the truth. Actually, it's one of those self-destructive beliefs, an illusion cultivated by social conditioning, that holds a lot of us men back from living happier, more fulfilled lives. In fact, when the heart is closed, there is suffering. There is fear and disconnection. When the heart is open, there is abundance. There is joy, vitality and love.

True, intelligent open-heartedness does not weaken you, it strengthens you. Heart-centred living means that you're more grounded, and less reactive. And within that lies your power. This is the stuff that makes a guy a great leader, a great dad, a good mate that you know that you can talk to and rely on. It's not about being overly sentimental or 'hippy-trippy' but about being emotionally intelligent and actually having clarity of mind.

Heart-centred men are able to step into their natural selves and to communicate with others from that more peaceful place; to hold compassionate boundaries and to respect other people's boundaries too.

When we live with an open heart, both on and off the yoga mat, we're able to access the full spectrum of emotions and express them from a place of authenticity, self-love and understanding. For example, uncontained, aggressive anger is often violent and destructive. Yet, with an open heart, you can look at your anger, process it and communicate it in a conscious, clear and effective way.

So how do you open your heart more? By hitting the yoga mat regularly, frequently integrating mindfulness practices like meditation and conscious breathing, and also being willing to explore your fundamental emotional truth. This is a process that can feel confrontational, uncomfortable and even painful, at times. Yet, in our experience, it's well worth it, leading you to true self-fulfilment and personal liberation.

Try these postures, which are designed to open the chest, shoulders and heart centre.

Bridge (see pp. 92–3)
Cobra (see pp. 104–5)
Cat/Cow (see pp. 42–3)
Extended Side Angle (see pp. 78–9)

THE YOGI WITHIN

We've all seen that yoga guy. He's skinny, bendy, long-limbed, long-haired, smells of bergamot, and talks like he's in an Eastern Philosophical cult. But is he a yogi?

A yogi is not defined by what he looks like (or smells like) or by how perfectly he executes his yoga poses. Rather, he's defined by his commitment to the practice, both on and off the mat. You can be any shape or size, nationality, age, fitness and flexibility level. Being a yogi isn't just about twisting and bending your body, it's also about applying the many principles of conscious living to all aspects of your life.

Here's the thing: a yogi is not something you become, but something you access. He's already within you, now, but it takes commitment and discipline to realise him.

So, who is this yogi? He's a seeker, curious to discover who he truly is. He has the desire to evolve; he wants to break through his masks, shadows and delusions, without fear. A yogi is truthful, authentic and very much real. He has compassion for himself and for all living creatures. This includes the environment.

A yogi is a man of good character. He is patient, gentle and kind; measured, calm and objective. He knows, too, that he is part of a great lineage (of yogis), and wishes to explore and pass on this wonderful ancient wisdom.

A yogi is a rich man. We don't mean money-rich (though perhaps he is that too); a yogi is 'rich' because he has a pure heart, good relationships and a healthy body.

Yoga is the tool for you to tap into all of that potential – potential that is already there, inside of you. There are many steps on the path to awakening your inner yogi. What's important is that you start walking them.

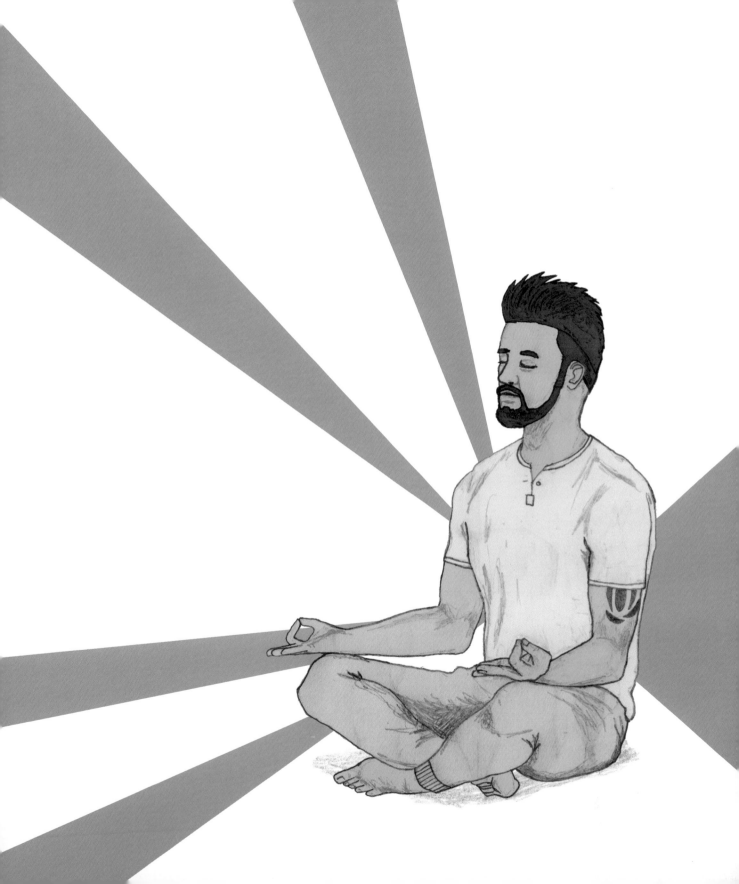

THE SEQUENCES

Now that we've introduced you to the various postures, breath practices and meditations, let's bring everything together. The following programme of five yoga sequences has been especially designed to help you progress from absolute beginner to confident yogi.

We suggest that you start with Sequence I. You'll find it gentle, accessible and a necessary foundation to the rest of the programme. Each sequence builds upon the previous one. As you master Sequence 1, you're ready for Sequence 2, and so on.

For best results, frequency is imperative. Make the commitment to get on your mat three to four times a week (even better if you do it every day).

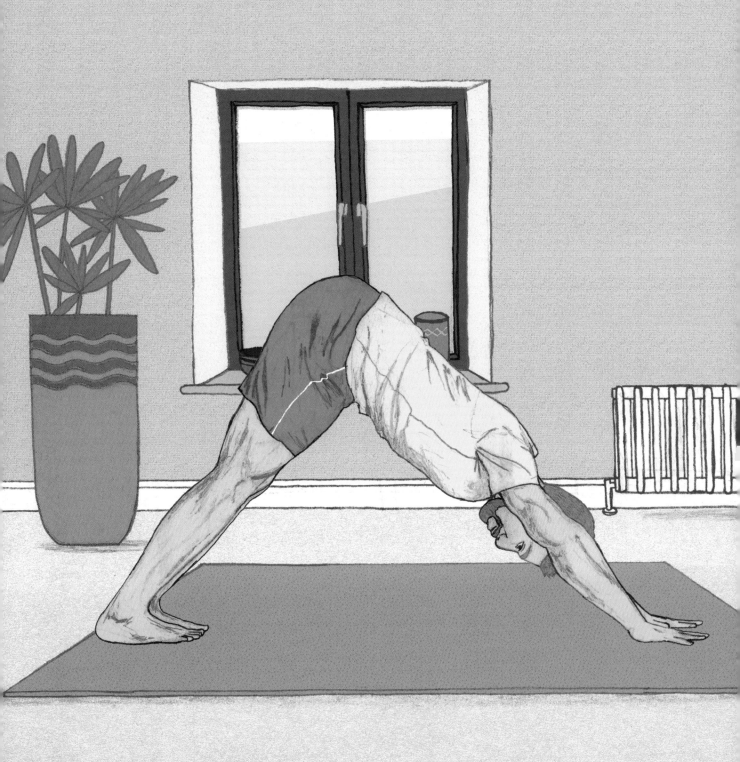

SEQUENCE 1

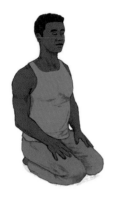

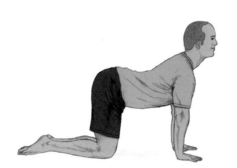

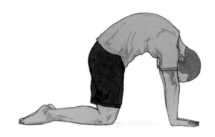

1 Easy Pose with Four-Part Breath
5 rounds of breath

2 Cow
Inhale

3 Cat
Exhale x 5 breaths

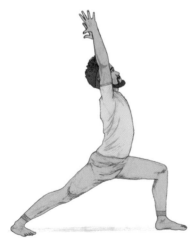

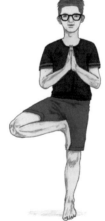

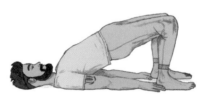

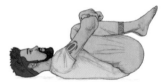

8 Warrior I
5 breaths – then return to Mountain Pose and repeat on opposite side

9 Tree Pose
5 breaths – then repeat on opposite side

10 Bridge
5 breaths

11 Wind-Relieving Pose
5 breaths

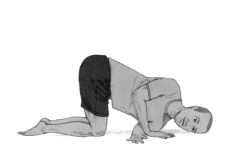
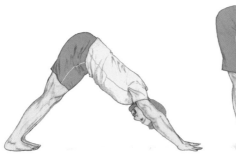
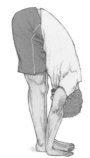
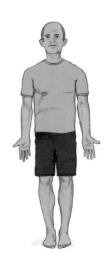

4 Thread the Needle
5 breaths – then repeat
on opposite side

5 Downward-Facing Dog
5 breaths – then
step to the front
of your mat

6 Standing Forward Fold
5 breaths – then
roll your spine up
to standing

7 Mountain Pose
5 breaths

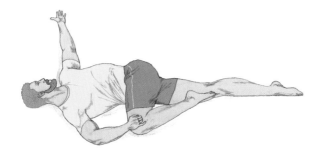
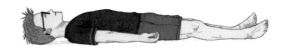

12 Supine Twist
5 breaths – then repeat on opposite side

13 Corpse
5 minutes

SEQUENCE 2

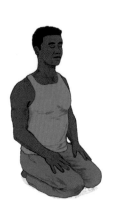

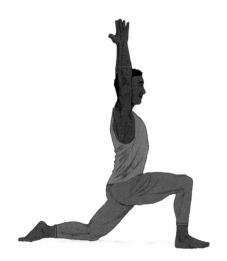

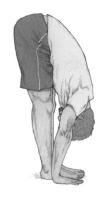

1 **Repeat Steps 1–5 from Sequence 1**

2 **Low Lunge**
5 breaths – then repeat on opposite side

3 **Standing Forward Fold**
5 breaths

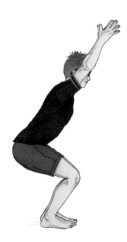

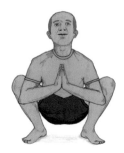

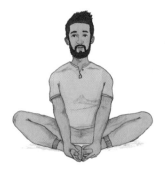

7 **Chair Pose**
5 breaths

8 **Garland**
5 breaths

9 **Butterfly**
5 breaths

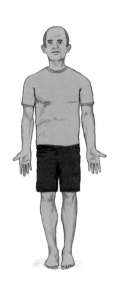

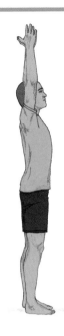

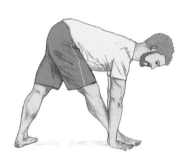

4   Mountain Pose
5 breaths

5   Sun Salutation A
1 to 3 rounds

6   Pyramid
5 breaths – then repeat
on opposite side

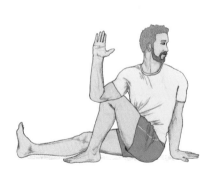

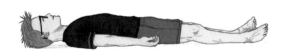

10   Seated Twist
5 breaths – then repeat
on opposite side

11   Corpse
5 minutes

SEQUENCE 3

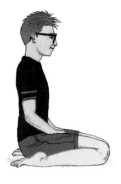

**1 Hero Pose with Alternate
Nostril Breathing**
5 rounds of breath

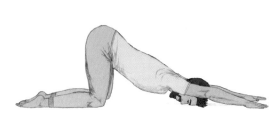

**2 Repeat Steps 2–4
from Sequence 1**

3 Puppy Pose
5 breaths

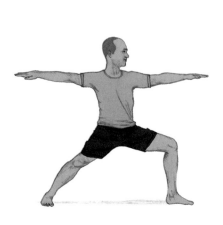

7 Warrior II
5 breaths

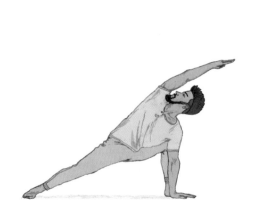

8 Extended Side Angle
5 breaths – then repeat
Steps 6–8 on opposite
side

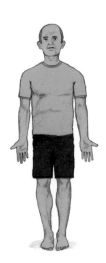

9 Mountain Pose
5 breaths

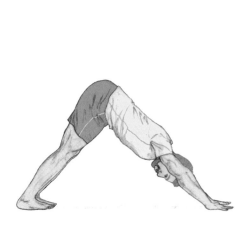

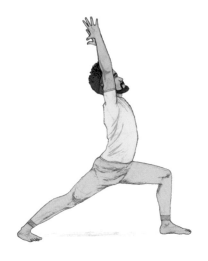

4 Downward-Facing Dog
5 breaths

5 Repeat Steps 2–5 from Sequence 2

6 Warrior I
5 breaths

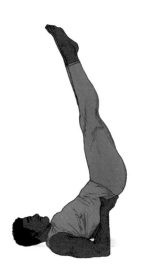

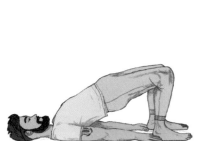

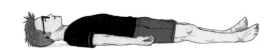

10 Repeat Steps 10–12 from Sequence 1

11 Half Shoulder Stand
5 breaths

12 Corpse
5 minutes

SEQUENCE 4

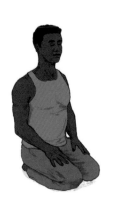
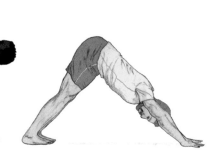
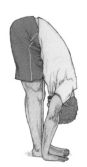

1 **Repeat Steps 1–4 from Sequence 1**

2 **Side Plank**
5 breaths – then repeat on opposite side

3 **Downward-Facing Dog**
5 breaths

4 **Standing Forward Fold**
5 breaths

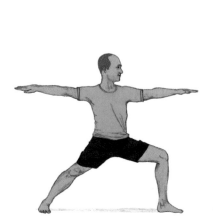
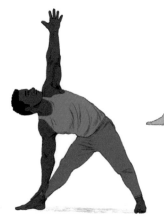
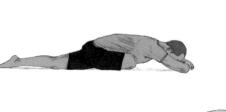

9 **Warrior II**
5 breaths

10 **Triangle**
5 breaths – then repeat Steps 8–11 on opposite side

11 **Pigeon**
5 breaths

12 **Head to Knee Forward Bend**
5 breaths

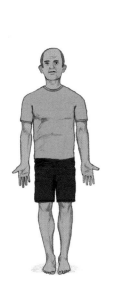
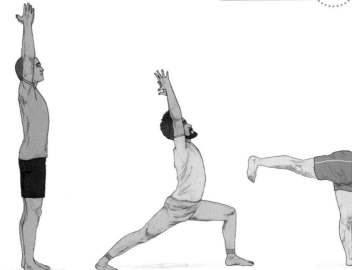

5 **Mountain Pose**
5 breaths

6 **Sun Salutation A**
1 to 3 rounds

7 **Warrior I**
5 breaths

8 **Warrior III**
5 breaths

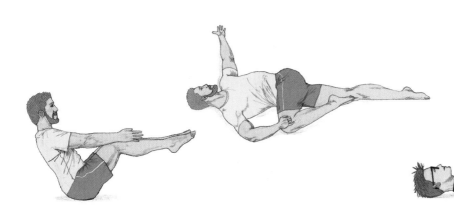

13 **Boat Pose**
5 breaths

14 **Supine Twist**
5 breaths – then repeat
on opposite side

15 **Corpse**
5 minutes

SEQUENCE 5

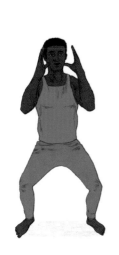

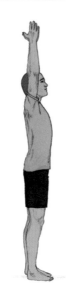

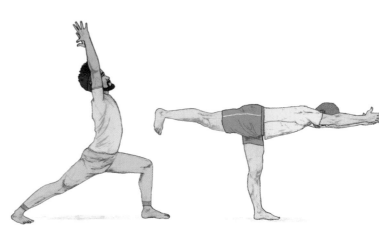

1 Warrior Breath
5 breaths

2 Sun Salutation A
1 to 3 rounds

3 Warrior I
5 breaths

4 Warrior III
5 breaths

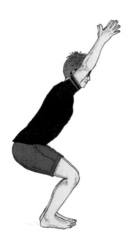

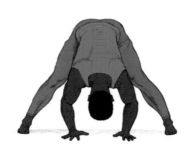

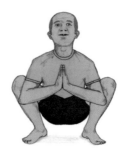

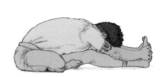

9 Chair Pose
5 breaths – then
repeat on left side

**10 Wide-Legged
Forward Fold**
5 breaths

11 Garland
5 breaths

**12 Repeat Steps
12 – 15 from
Sequence 4**

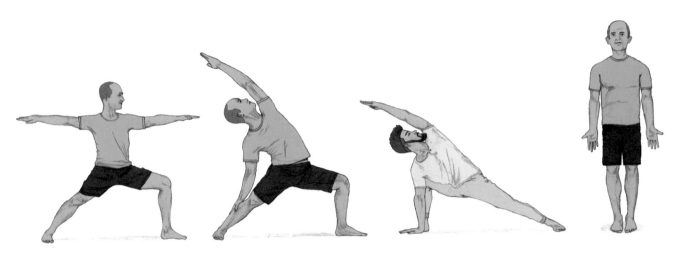

5 Warrior II
5 breaths

6 Reverse Warrior
5 breaths

**7 Extended Side
Angle**
5 breaths

8 Mountain Pose
5 breaths – then
repeat Steps 3–8
on opposite side

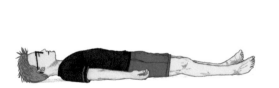

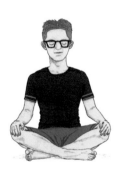

13 Corpse
5 minutes

**14 Meditation:
Lightness of Being**
5 minutes

Jarod's story

My story is a marvellous demonstration of the lasting power of yoga through the months, years and decades of a man's life. Now in my early fifties, I first hit the mat aged 18. It was back in Sydney, Australia, when yoga was neither as popular nor accessible as it is today, and I went because I was curious – about the philosophy, more than the postures – having already discovered the brilliance of endorphins, via running, cycling and dancing.

What I needed now was guidance. I was a spiritually open young man with a wild and loving nature but losing my mother, when I was 22, was a huge and unexpected blow that sent me spinning off the mat and towards harder, faster hobbies that could numb my grief in minutes. But self-medicating with alcohol and other mind-altering substances is hardly a long-term solution is it, guys? Soon enough I returned to yoga. I fell in love with it again. Then out of love with it. Then in. Again, again, again. Me and yoga, we might say, have been married and divorced a few times over. Yet the love just kept returning, deeper and more profound each time. From the fiendishly challenging practice of Ashtanga yoga, which requires 90 minutes practice (minimum) per day in its basic form, to long discussions with spiritual leaders and the intense discipline of silent retreat – I tried it all.

Then, at last, when in my forties, I met Caleb, a yoga teacher who walked the walk and talked the talk. We two became close friends and, slowly but surely, Caleb re-inspired and encouraged me to return to yoga and stick with it. In the midst of this, together we created a platform for sharing the ancient practice and philosophy of yoga for the modern day man. And so, Wellness Warrior was born.

Yoga is the perfect addition to my existing fitness schedule, which is full of cycling, running and strength training. It is, for the recreational athlete (or any active person with training goals), a true barometer of where the body is at; each posture offering information as to what is stiff, weak, tight or strong. Not only do the postures help to ease out hamstring, quad and back stiffness but they also enable me to tap back into what I call 'the field of pure consciousness' – a space that is full of creative and spiritual potential and which, I can now see, was what I was searching for all along.

When things go awry, physically, mentally, emotionally or spiritually, I know where I must go. Always to the mat. Sun salutations, chanting and the breath. These are the things that ground me and steer me. Back to the practice. To my values. To myself. These days the mat is less a place where I go searching and more a place where I come home. Never stop returning is the message. And one day I won't leave.

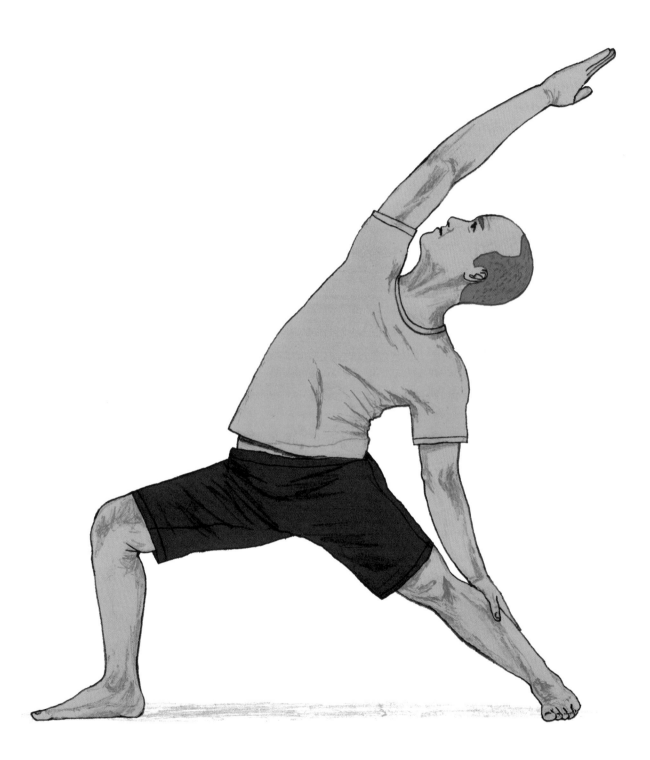

GLOSSARY

COMMONLY USED YOGA TERMS

Asana
The postures; the physical practice of yoga.

Chakra
In Sanskrit 'chakra' translates to 'wheel' and refers to the seven main energy centres in the body.

Connected breath
The practice of deep and conscious breathing while maintaining a posture.

Engaged core
To brace all the muscles in your torso while maintaining a stable breath.

Extension
The action where you increase the angle of a joint, such as straightening your knees.

Flexion
The action where you decrease the angle of a joint, such as flexion of the foot at the ankle.

Fold
To lengthen your torso over your thighs.

Glutes
The nickname given to the group of muscles that make up your buttocks.

Hip flexors
The muscle group at the top of your thighs that enables you to bend at the waist and lift your knees up.

Hips square
To position your hips in the same plane, both vertically and horizontally.

Hyperextension
The extension or straightening of any joint beyond its normal range of motion.

Lengthened spine
Gently stretching the spinal muscles and ligaments to create space between the vertebrae.

Neutral spine
The natural position of the spine where your pelvis, ribcage and skull are in alignment with each other.

Release
Deepening into a posture as you exhale.

Sacrum
The shield-shaped bone at the base of your lumbar vertebrae that holds your spine and pelvis together.

Sanskrit
The ancient Indian language that was spoken by the first yogis.

Sit bones
Your sit bones are the boney bumps located in the flesh of your buttock. Anatomically, they are part of the pelvis.

Stacking
Where joints are vertically aligned allowing you to use your strength more effectively with less strain.

Tailbone
This is the last bone at the base of your spine above your buttocks. It is officially called the coccyx.

Third Eye
The sixth chakra, located in the centre of your forehead, considered to be your mind's eye.

Tucked pelvis
Where you gently roll the pubic bone towards the ribcage to flatten the lower back curve.

Yogi
A person who regularly practices yoga.

ANATOMY

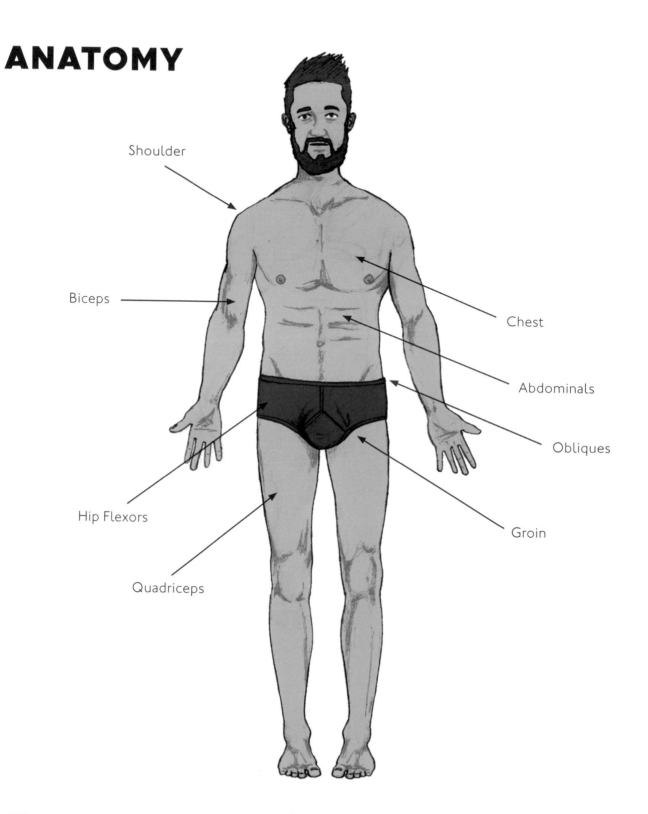

Shoulder

Biceps

Chest

Abdominals

Obliques

Hip Flexors

Groin

Quadriceps

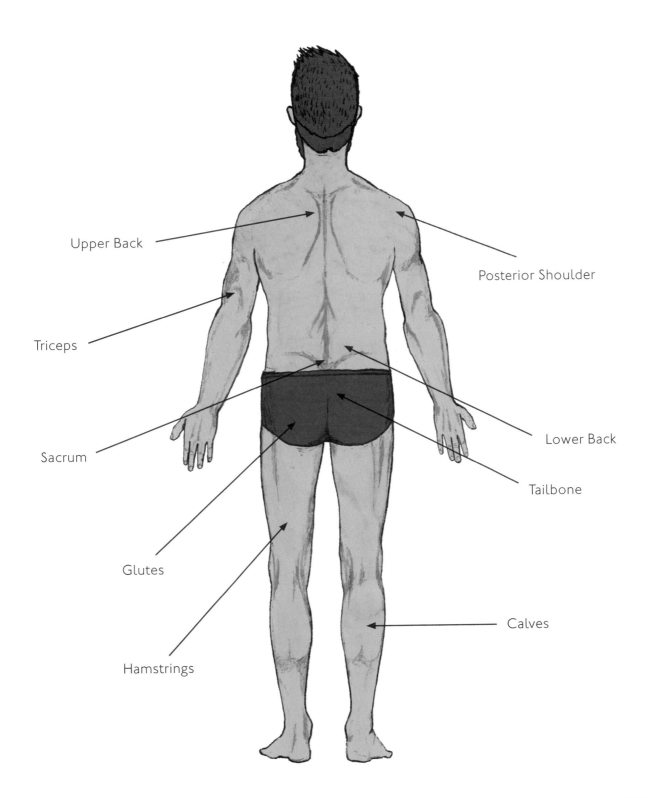

Upper Back

Posterior Shoulder

Triceps

Sacrum

Lower Back

Tailbone

Glutes

Hamstrings

Calves

ABOUT THE AUTHORS

Caleb Jude Packham is an Australian TV presenter turned internationally renowned yoga teacher. He is committed to making yoga accessible to all – particularly men. He has staged large-scale yoga events in iconic London venues, and taught extensively on the international yoga circuit. In 2018 he co-founded Wellness Warrior, a multi-channel yoga brand delivering physical, mental and emotional fitness.

@calebjudepackhamyoga

Jarod Chapman is a health and wellbeing expert and co-founder of Wellness Warrior. He is the former personal wellness coach to Tina Turner and media ambassador for Bio Medical Research Ltd. As a wellness writer he has contributed to the UK's bestselling magazines and regularly appears on UK and European radio.

@jarod.chapman

www.wellnesswarrior.yoga

ACKNOWLEDGEMENTS

This book would not be possible without our amazing team of family, friends and creatives.

A big shout out and thank you to our editors, Charlotte Croft and Zoë Blanc, and the Bloomsbury crew for guiding us and believing in our mission to inspire more men onto the yoga mat.

To our agents, Nick Walters and David Luxton, thank you for championing us all the way.

To Lucy Fry, your support has been immeasurable.

To David Broadbent, thank you for bringing our book to life through the character and humanity of your illustrations.

To Sara Bellamy, for your vision and generosity.

A big thank you to Luke Lloyd-Davies for your belief in us – you've certainly made some dreams come true.

To Anand Mehrotra and the Sattva Yoga Academy - thank you for your inspirational teachings.

And special thanks to this lot (and each of you know why):
Jimmy Alfred, Graham Bartlett, Peter Cashmore, Min Carroll, Scott, Lisa & Debra Chapman, Susie Clements, Tim & Colleen Crescenti, Urtema Dolphin, John Gibson, Carrie Ann Huddleston, Sarah Jordan, Eddie McAteer, Caroline, Donna & Roger Packham, Antonio Peixoto, Rebecca Rainbow, Leila Sadeghee, Lourdes Santin, Mike Small, Mark Wakeling, Darren Walsh, Jez Smith and Kylie Watson.

And lastly, thank you to all of the men who've joined our ever expanding tribe of warriors. Let's keep growing this movement together.

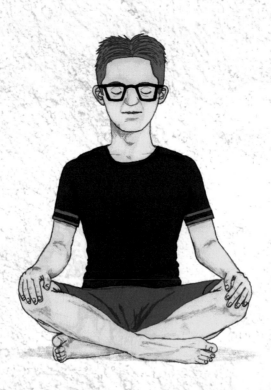

This book is dedicated to our mums and
all of the great women in our lives.